Changing Landscape of Heart Failure Imaging

Editor

PURVI PARWANI

HEART FAILURE CLINICS

www.heartfailure.theclinics.com

Consulting Editor
EDUARDO BOSSONE

Founding Editor
JAGAT NARULA

October 2023 • Volume 19 • Number 4

ELSEVIER

1600 John F. Kennedy Boulevard • Suite 1800 • Philadelphia, Pennsylvania, 19103-2899

http://www.theclinics.com

HEART FAILURE CLINICS Volume 19, Number 4
October 2023 ISSN 1551-7136, ISBN-13: 978-0-443-18314-0

Editor: Joanna Gascoine
Developmental Editor: Nitesh Barthwal

Heart Failure Clinics (ISSN 1551-7136) is published quarterly by Elsevier Inc., 360 Park Avenue South, New York, NY 10010-1710. Months of publication are January, April, July, and October. Business and editorial offices: 1600 John F. Kennedy Boulevard, Suite 1800, Philadelphia, PA 19103-2899. Periodicals postage paid at New York, NY, and additional mailing offices. Subscription prices are USD 291.00 per year for US individuals, USD 629.00 per year for US institutions, USD 100.00 per year for US students and residents, USD 315.00 per year for Canadian individuals, USD 729.00 per year for Canadian institutions, USD 331.00 per year for international individuals, USD 729.00 per year for international institutions, and USD 100.00 per year for Canadian and foreign students/residents. To receive student and resident rate, orders must be accompanied by name of affiliated institution, date of term, and the *signature* of program/residency coordinator on institution letterhead. Orders will be billed at individual rate until proof of status is received. Foreign air speed delivery is included in all *Clinics* subscription prices. All prices are subject to change without notice. **POSTMASTER:** Send address changes to *Heart Failure Clinics*, Elsevier Health Sciences Division, Subscription Customer Service, 3251 Riverport Lane, Maryland Heights, MO 63043. **Customer Service: 1-800-654-2452 (US and Canada). From outside of the US and Canada, call 314-447-8871. Fax: 314-447-8029. For print support, E-mail: JournalsCustomerService-usa@elsevier.com. For online support, E-mail: JournalsOnlineSupport-usa@elsevier.com.**

Reprints. For copies of 100 or more of articles in this publication, please contact the Commercial Reprints Department, Elsevier Inc., 360 Park Avenue South, New York, NY 10010-1710. Tel.: 212-633-3874; Fax: 212-633-3820; E-mail: reprints@elsevier.com.

Heart Failure Clinics is covered in *MEDLINE/PubMed (Index Medicus).*

Contributors

CONSULTING EDITOR

EDUARDO BOSSONE, MD, PhD, FCCP, FESC, FACC
Consulting Editor, *Heart Failure Clinics*, Director of Cardiology, Cardarelli Hospital, Department of Public Health, Department of Translational Medical Sciences, University of Naples "Federico II," Naples, Italy

EDITOR

PURVI PARWANI, MBBS, MPH, FACC
Associate Professor of Medicine, Multimodality Cardiovascular Imager, Division of Cardiology, Department of Medicine, Loma Linda University Health, Loma Linda, California, USA

AUTHORS

GUPTA AAKASH, MD
Division of Cardiology, Department of Medicine, Loma Linda University Health, Loma Linda, California, USA

DMITRY ABRAMOV, MD
Assistant Professor of Medicine, Division of Cardiology, Loma Linda University Medical Center, Loma Linda University Health, Loma Linda, California, USA

VRATIKA AGARWAL, MD
Division of Cardiology, Department of Medicine, Columbia University Irving Medical Center, NewYork-Presbyterian Hospital, New York, New York, USA

AMRO ALSAID, MD, FSCMR
Medical Director, Cardiac MRI and Cardiac CT Labs, Department of Cardiology, Baylor Scott & White The Heart Hospital, Plano, Texas, USA

SENTHIL S. BALASUBRAMANIAN, MD
Division of Cardiology, Montefiore Medical Center, Albert Einstein College of Medicine, Bronx, New York, USA; Division of Cardiology, University of Chicago at Northshore University Health System, Evanston, Illinois, USA

GIULIO BALESTRIERI, MD
Cardiology Unit, Hospital Papa Giovanni XXIII, Bergamo, Italy

DHRUBAJYOTI BANDYOPADHYAY, MD
Department of Cardiology, New York Medical College, Westchester Medical Center, Valhalla, New York, USA

SOHAIB AHMAD BASHARAT, MD
Fellow-in-Training, Division of Cardiology, Loma Linda University Medical Center, Loma Linda, California, USA

ANTONI BAYES-GENIS, MD, PhD
Department of Cardiology, Heart Institute, University Hospital Germans Trias i Pujol, ICREC Research Program, Germans Trias i Pujol Health Science Research Institute, Badalona, Spain; CIBER Cardiovascular, Madrid, Spain; Department of Medicine, Autonomous University of Barcelona, Barcelona, Spain

ANDREW J. BRADLEY, MD
Division of Cardiology, Department of
Medicine, The George Washington University
School of Medicine and Health Sciences,
Washington, DC, USA

ANDREW D. CHOI, MD
Division of Cardiology, Department of
Medicine, The George Washington University
School of Medicine and Health Sciences,
Washington, DC, USA

MICHELA GIOVANNA COCCIA, MD
Cardiology Unit, Voghera Hospital, ASST
Pavia, Voghera, Italy

PEDRO COVAS, MD
Division of Cardiology, Department of
Medicine, The George Washington University
School of Medicine and Health Sciences,
Washington, DC, USA

EMILIA D'ELIA, MD, PhD, FESC
Cardiology Unit, Hospital Papa Giovanni XXIII,
Bergamo, Italy

SALVATORE D'ISA, MD
Cardiology Unit, Hospital Papa Giovanni XXIII,
Bergamo, Italy

VICTORIA DELGADO, MD, PhD
Cardiovascular Imaging Section, Department
of Cardiology, Heart Institute, University
Hospital Germans Trias i Pujol, Centre de
Medicina Comparativa i Bioimatge, Badalona,
Spain

ADITYA DESAI, MD
Department of Internal Medicine, University of
California Riverside School of Medicine,
Riverside, California, USA

DARSHI DESAI, MD
Department of Internal Medicine, University of
California Riverside School of Medicine,
Riverside, California, USA

BRIAN DIEP, MD
Division of Cardiology, Department of
Medicine, Loma Linda University Health, Loma
Linda, California, USA

MARIANNA FONTANA, MD, PhD
Director of the UCL CMR Unit at the Royal
Free Hospital, Professor of Cardiology, UCL
CMR Department at the Royal Free Hospital
and the National Amyloidosis Centre,
University College, London, United
Kingdom

MATTHIAS G. FRIEDRICH, MD
Professor of Medicine, Departments of
Medicine and Diagnostic Radiology, McGill
University Health Centre, Montreal, Quebec,
Canada

ANTHON FUISZ, MD, FACC
Department of Cardiology, New York Medical
College, Westchester Medical Center, Valhalla,
New York, USA

MARIO J. GARCIA, MD
Division of Cardiology, Montefiore Medical
Center, Albert Einstein College of Medicine,
Bronx, New York, USA

JALAJ GARG, MD, FESC
Cardiac Electrophysiologist, Assistant
Professor of Medicine, Division of Cardiology,
Loma Linda University Medical Center, Loma
Linda, California, USA

SAFWAN GAZNABI, MD
Division of Cardiology, Montefiore Medical
Center, Albert Einstein College of Medicine,
Bronx, New York, USA; Division of Cardiology,
University of Chicago at Northshore
University Health System, Evanston, Illinois,
USA

MALIK GHAWANMEH, MD
Division of Cardiology, Department of
Medicine, The George Washington University
School of Medicine and Health Sciences,
Washington, DC, USA

CARLOS A. GONGORA, MD
Division of Cardiology, Montefiore Medical
Center, Albert Einstein College of Medicine,
Bronx, New York, USA

ASHLEY M. GOVI, MD
Division of Cardiology, Department of
Medicine, The George Washington University
School of Medicine and Health Sciences,
Washington, DC, USA

REBECCA HAHN, MD
Division of Cardiology, Department of Medicine, Columbia University Irving Medical Center, NewYork-Presbyterian Hospital, New York, New York, USA

ADRIJA HAJRA, MD, MRCP
Department of Internal Medicine, Montefiore Medical Center, Albert Einstein College of Medicine, Bronx, New York, USA

EDWIN C. HO, MD
Division of Cardiology, Montefiore Medical Center, Albert Einstein College of Medicine, Bronx, New York, USA

INGRID HSIUNG, MD
Fellow-in-Training, Department of Cardiology, Baylor Scott & White The Heart Hospital, Plano, Texas, USA

NICOLAS KANG, MD
Internal Medicine Resident, Department of Medicine, Loma Linda University Medical Center, Loma Linda, California, USA

GIZEM KASA, MD
Cardiovascular Imaging Section, Department of Cardiology, Heart Institute, University Hospital Germans Trias i Pujol, Centre de Medicina Comparativa i Bioimatge, Badalona, Spain

CHRISTOPHER KRAMER, MD
Cardiovascular Division, Departments of Medicine, and Radiology and Medical Imaging, University of Virginia Health, Charlottesville, Virginia, USA

SURAJ KRISHNAN, MD
Department of Internal Medicine, Jacobi Hospital, Albert Einstein College of Medicine, Bronx, New York, USA

AZEEM LATIB, MD
Division of Cardiology, Montefiore Medical Center, Albert Einstein College of Medicine, Bronx, New York, USA

RAUL LIMONTA, MD
School of Medicine and Surgery, Milano Bicocca University, Milano, Italy

DANIEL LORENZATTI, MD
Division of Cardiology, Montefiore Medical Center, Albert Einstein College of Medicine, Bronx, New York, USA

ROBERTA MAGNANO, MD
Cardiology Unit, Hospital Santo Spirito, Pescara, Italy

THOMAS MAHER, MD
Department of Medicine, Morristown Medical Center, Morristown, New Jersey, USA

ANA MARTINEZ-NAHARRO, MD
UCL CMR Department at the Royal Free Hospital and the National Amyloidosis Centre, University College, London, United Kingdom

JEIRYM MIRANDA, MD
Division of Cardiology, Montefiore Medical Center, Albert Einstein College of Medicine, Bronx, New York, USA; Division of Cardiology, Mount Sinai, Morningside, New York, USA

ZACHARIAH NEALY, MD
Cardiovascular Division, Department of Medicine, University of Virginia Health, Charlottesville, Virginia, USA

GURUSHER PANJRATH, MD
Division of Cardiology, Department of Medicine, The George Washington University School of Medicine and Health Sciences, Washington, DC, USA

PURVI PARWANI, MBBS, MPH, FACC
Associate Professor of Medicine, Multimodality Cardiovascular Imager, Division of Cardiology, Department of Medicine, Loma Linda University Health, Loma Linda, California, USA

PAMELA PIÑA, MD
Division of Cardiology, Montefiore Medical Center, Albert Einstein College of Medicine, Bronx, New York, USA; Division of Cardiology, CEDIMAT, Santo Domingo, Dominican Republic

PRAGYA RANJAN, MD, FACC
Department of Cardiology, New York Medical College, Westchester Medical Center, Valhalla, New York, USA

ALDO L. SCHENONE, MD
Division of Cardiology, Montefiore Medical
Center, Albert Einstein College of Medicine,
Bronx, New York, USA

EDOARDO SCIATTI, MD
Cardiology Unit, Hospital Papa Giovanni XXIII,
Bergamo, Italy

ANDREA SCOTTI, MD
Division of Cardiology, Montefiore Medical
Center, Albert Einstein College of Medicine,
Bronx, New York, USA

RISHI SHRIVASTAV, MD
Department of Cardiology, Icahn School of
Medicine at Mount Sinai, Mount Sinai

Morningside Hospital, Cardiovascular Institute,
New York, New York, USA

LEANDRO SLIPCZUK, MD, PhD, FACC
Division of Cardiology, Montefiore Medical
Center, Albert Einstein College of Medicine,
Bronx, New York, USA

SETH URETSKY, MD, FACC, FSCMR, FASNC
Department of Cardiovascular Medicine,
Gagnon Cardiovascular Institute, Morristown
Medical Center, Atlantic Health System,
Morristown, New Jersey, USA

ANDREA VEGH, MD
Department of Medicine, Morristown Medical
Center, Morristown, New Jersey, USA

Contents

Heart failure (HF), a challenging and heterogeneous syndrome, still remains a major health problem worldwide, despite all the advances in prevention, diagnosis, and treatment of cardiovascular disease. Cardiac imaging plays a pivotal role in the classification of HF, accurate diagnosis of underlying etiology and decision-making. Integration of other imaging techniques such as cardiac magnetic resonance, nuclear imaging, and exercise imaging testing is important to characterize HF accurately. This article reviews the role of multimodality imaging to diagnose patients with HF.

A multimodality imaging evaluation in hypertrophic cardiomyopathy is often used for risk stratification. Recent developments in imaging have allowed for better diagnosis, prognosis, and decision-making for a variety of therapies from medical to interventional. Echocardiography and magnetic resonance have been integral in evaluating subtype, left ventricular function, tissue characterization, left atrial measurements, valvular function, and presence of left ventricular aneurysm and outflow tract obstruction. These factors have helped to quantify risk of atrial fibrillation and determine the likely usefulness of pharmacologic therapy and septal reduction therapy. This review covers these in detail.

Arrhythmogenic cardiomyopathy (ACM) is an umbrella term encompassing a wide variety of overlapping hereditary and nonhereditary disorders that can result in malignant ventricular arrhythmias and sudden cardiac death. Cardiac MRI plays a critical role in accurate diagnosis of various ACM entities and is increasingly showing promise in risk stratification that can further guide management particularly in decisions regarding use of implantable cardioverter defibrillator. Genotyping plays an important role in cascade testing but challenges remain due to incomplete penetrance and wide phenotypic variability of ACM as well as the presence of gene-elusive cases.

Advancements in quantitative cardiac magnetic resonance (CMR) have revolutionized the diagnosis and management of viral myocarditis. With the addition of T1 and T2 mapping parameters in the updated Lake Louise Criteria, CMR can diagnose myocarditis with superior diagnostic accuracy compared with endomyocardial biopsy, especially in stable patients. Additionally, the unique value of CMR tissue characterization continues to improve the diagnosis and risk stratification of myocarditis. This review will discuss new and ongoing developments in cardiovascular imaging and its application to noninvasive diagnosis, prognostication, and management of viral myocarditis and its complications.

Edoardo Sciatti, Michela Giovanna Coccia, Roberta Magnano, Gupta Aakash, Raul Limonta, Brian Diep, Giulio Balestrieri, Salvatore D'Isa, Dmitry Abramov, Purvi Parwani, and Emilia D'Elia

While the prevalence of heart failure, in general, is similar in men and women, women experience a higher rate of HFpEF compared to HFrEF. Cardiovascular risk factors, parity, estrogen levels, cardiac physiology, and altered response to the immune system may be at the root of this difference. Studies have found that in response to increasing age and hypertension, women experience more concentric left ventricle remodeling, more ventricular and arterial stiffness, and less ventricular dilation compared to men, which predisposes women to developing more diastolic dysfunction. A multi-modality imaging approach is recommended to identify patients with HFpEF. Particularly, appreciation of sex-based differences as described in this review is important in optimizing the evaluation and care of women with HFpEF.

Rishi Shrivastav, Adrija Hajra, Suraj Krishnan, Dhrubajyoti Bandyopadhyay, Pragya Ranjan, and Anthon Fuisz

A high clinical suspicion in the setting of appropriate history, physical exam, laboratory, and imaging parameters is often required to set the groundwork for diagnosis and management. Echocardiography may show septal thinning, evidence of systolic and diastolic dysfunction, along with impaired global longitudinal strain. Cardiac MRI reveals late gadolinium enhancement along with evidence of myocardial edema and inflammation on T2 weighted imaging and parametric mapping. 18F-FDG PET detects the presence of active inflammation and the presence of scar. Involvement of the right ventricle on MRI or PET confers a high risk for adverse cardiac events and mortality.

Safwan Gaznabi, Jeirym Miranda, Daniel Lorenzatti, Pamela Piña, Senthil S. Balasubramanian, Darshi Desai, Aditya Desai, Edwin C. Ho, Andrea Scotti, Carlos A. Gongora, Aldo L. Schenone, Mario J. Garcia, Azeem Latib, Purvi Parwani, and Leandro Slipczuk

Current guidelines of aortic stenosis (AS) management focus on valve parameters, LV systolic dysfunction, and symptoms; however, emerging data suggest that there may be benefit of aortic valve replacement before it becomes severe by present criteria. Myocardial assessment using novel multimodality imaging techniques exhibits subclinical myocardial injury and remodeling at various stages before guideline-directed interventions, which predicts adverse outcomes. This raises the question of whether implementing serial myocardial assessment should become part of the standard appraisal, thereby identifying high-risk patients aiming to minimize adverse outcomes.

Vratika Agarwal and Rebecca Hahn

During the last few years, there has been a substantial shift in efforts to understand and manage secondary or functional tricuspid regurgitation (TR) given its prevalence, adverse prognostic impact, and symptom burden associated with progressive right heart failure. Understanding the pathophysiology of TR and right heart failure is crucial for determining the best treatment strategy and improving outcomes. In this article, we review the complex relationship between right heart structural and hemodynamic changes that drive the pathophysiology of secondary TR and discuss the role of multi-modality imaging in the diagnosis, management, and determination of outcomes.

Mitral regurgitation is a common valvular heart disease with increasing prevalence due to the aging population. In degenerative (primary) mitral regurgitation, medical therapies are limited and the mainstay of treatment is mitral valve surgery. Patients are referred for mitral valve surgery based on the American College of Cardiology/ American Heart Association guidelines, which recommend surgery in patients with severe mitral regurgitation. Echocardiography uses multiple parameters that lack re-producibility and accuracy. Studies comparing cardiovascular magnetic resonance (CMR) and echocardiography have shown that CMR is a better predictor of clinical outcome and postsurgical left ventricular remodeling than echocardiography.

Artificial intelligence (AI) applications are expanding in cardiac imaging. AI research has shown promise in workflow optimization, disease diagnosis, and integration of clinical and imaging data to predict patient outcomes. The diagnostic and prognostic paradigm of heart failure is heavily reliant on cardiac imaging. As AI becomes increasingly validated and integrated into clinical practice, AI influence on heart failure management will grow. This review discusses areas of current research and potential clinical applications in AI as applied to heart failure cardiac imaging.

HEART FAILURE CLINICS

SERIES OF RELATED INTEREST

Cardiology Clinics
http://www.cardiology.theclinics.com/
Cardiac Electrophysiology Clinics
https://www.cardiacep.theclinics.com/
Interventional Cardiology Clinics
https://www.interventional.theclinics.com/

THE CLINICS ARE AVAILABLE ONLINE!
Access your subscription at:
www.theclinics.com

Preface
Changing Landscape of Heart Failure Imaging

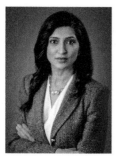 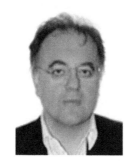

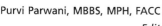

Purvi Parwani, MBBS, MPH, FACC   Eduardo Bossone, MD, PhD
Editors

There are approximately 825,000 new cases of heart failure (HF) that occur just in the United States every year. This number is expected to exceed 8 million new cases by the year 2030. Currently, approximately 6.7 million Americans $\geq$20 years of age have HF.[1] Diagnosis of HF remains complex and heterogenous; however, correct diagnosis leads to accurate treatment and possibly a decrease in patient morbidity and mortality. Advanced imaging, mainly, cardiovascular magnetic resonance imaging, coronary computed tomography angiography, and nuclear imaging like PET, has progressed significantly in last few decades. With the advent of new imaging technologies, phenotyping the patients with HF has become easier. A clinician treating a patient with HF must possess knowledge about various indications for use of multimodality imaging. Even if the diagnosis is made, staging or severity of the disease and prognostication might require use of various noninvasive imaging modalities.[2] The present issue focuses on the use of novel imaging modalities to assess the disease status, severity, and underlying pathophysiology to determine the correct diagnosis and further to prognosticate the patients.

In this special issue, we discuss the change in the paradigm of HF imaging by providing the latest updates in multimodality imaging. We discuss the role of advanced imaging in patients with cardiac sarcoidosis and hypertrophic cardiomyopathy beyond the risk stratification. We provide deeper insight into diagnosis of viral myocarditis and resultant dilated cardiomyopathy, especially incorporating the learning from COVID myocarditis literature. Basharat and colleagues and Bradley and colleagues dive deep into the complex decision-making process for patients with imaging characteristic for arrhythmogenic cardiomyopathy with various clinical phenotypic manifestations. In the recent years, literature has made it evident that heart failure preserved ejection fraction (HFpEF) is a complex heterogenous spectrum of disease. Delia and colleagues further discuss this and sex differences that exist with the diagnosis of HFpEF. Even though echocardiography remains the main imaging modality for the evaluation of patients with valvular heart disease, further technological and other advances in advanced imaging now have provided a novel insight into pathophysiology and quantification based on prognostic assessment. This is further explored in the article focusing on the advanced imaging assessment of aortic stenosis, tricuspid regurgitation, and mitral regurgitation. Finally, Bradley and colleagues and Choi and colleagues provide a fantastic review of the emerging role of artificial intelligence in HF imaging.

Heart Failure Clin 19 (2023) xi–xii
https://doi.org/10.1016/j.hfc.2023.06.005
1551-7136/23/© 2023 Published by Elsevier Inc.

I thank all the authors for their valuable insights and contributions to this novel and unique issue.

Purvi Parwani, MBBS, MPH, FACC
Division of Cardiology
Department of medicine
Loma Linda University Health
Loma Linda, CA, USA

Eduardo Bossone, MD, PhD
Department of Public Health
Department of Translational Medical Sciences
University of Naples "Federico II"
Ed. 18, I piano, Via Sergio Pansini 5
Naples 80131, Italy

E-mail addresses:
drpurviparwani@gmail.com (P. Parwani)
eduardo.bossone@unina.it (E. Bossone)

REFERENCES

1. Tsao CW, Aday AW, Almarzooq ZI, et al. Heart disease and stroke statistics—2023 update: a report from the American Heart Association. Circulation 2023;147(8):e93–621.
2. Adigopula S, Grapsa J. Advances in imaging and heart failure: where are we heading? Card Fail Rev 2018;4(2):73–7.

Latest Updates in Heart Failure Imaging

Gizem Kasa, MD, Antoni Bayes-Genis, MD, PhD, Victoria Delgado, MD, PhD*

KEYWORDS

- Multimodality imaging • Heart failure • Echocardiography • Cardiac magnetic resonance

KEY POINTS

- Cardiac imaging plays a crucial role in the accurate diagnosis of heart failure (HF).
- Echocardiography is commonly used as the initial imaging technique, with left ventricular ejection fraction (LVEF) being the main parameter for classification of HF and risk stratification.
- LVEF alone is not sufficient to diagnose the HF etiology and personalize the decision-making. In the most contemporary HF guidelines, the need to integrate novel cardiac function measurements, such as evaluation of left ventricular diastolic function and myocardial deformation, has been highlighted.
- Multimodality imaging, especially cardiac magnetic resonance with myocardial tissue characterization, is key to diagnose etiology of HF and provides incremental prognostic value.

INTRODUCTION

Heart failure (HF) is a complex clinical syndrome. Symptoms occur when structural and/or functional abnormality of the heart results in elevated intracardiac pressures and/or inadequate cardiac output. Despite major therapeutical advances, HF remains a major public health problem. Due to the population growth, aging, and the increasing prevalence of comorbidities, the absolute number of hospital admissions for HF is expected to increase considerably in the future.[1,2] Identifying the cause of HF is important because each cause may require specific treatment. Cardiac imaging has a crucial role in the classification of HF and the accurate diagnosis of the underlying cause.

Phenotyping of HF is the first approach to classify patients with HF symptoms and initiate treatment. For decades, this classification has been based on left ventricular ejection fraction (LVEF) measures. Although randomized clinical trials have shown efficacy of HF medical and device-based therapies in patients with LVEF 40% or lesser,[3] the efficacy of new specific medical therapies in patients with mildly reduced or preserved LVEF has not been demonstrated until recently.[4,5] Participant-level data analysis from recent randomized clinical trials has shown that the benefits of combining mineralocorticoid receptor antagonists, angiotensin-receptor neprilysin inhibitor, and sodium-glucose cotransporter 2 inhibitors extended up to an LVEF of 65%, questioning the usefulness of HF classification based on this functional parameter.[6] In addition, phenotyping HF with LVEF may not be enough, particularly if we aim to detect subclinical left ventricular (LV) systolic dysfunction in population at risk of HF (Stages A and B) and prevent the occurrence of clinically symptomatic HF.

The latest American College of Cardiology (ACC)/American Heart Association (AHA) and the European Society of Cardiology (ESC) guidelines maintain the LVEF-based HF classification; however, there is clear emphasis on adding new objective measures such as the evidence of increased LV filling pressures in patients with HF with mildly reduced EF (HFmrEF) and HF with preserved EF (HFpEF). In this regard, exercise stress testing and echocardiographic evaluation of diastolic parameters are of importance. Furthermore, the

Cardiovascular Imaging Section, Department of Cardiology, Heart Institute, University Hospital Germans Trias i Pujol, Badalona, Spain
* Corresponding author. Carretera de Canyet s/n, Badalona 08916, Barcelona.
E-mail address: vdelgadog.germanstrias@gencat.cat

Heart Failure Clin 19 (2023) 407–418
https://doi.org/10.1016/j.hfc.2023.03.007
1551-7136/23/© 2023 Elsevier Inc. All rights reserved.

heartfailure.theclinics.com

incremental value of myocardial deformation parameters, such as global longitudinal strain (GLS), to predict the risk of developing HF or recurrent HF hospitalizations is also highlighted. The use of natriuretic peptides is also recommended in the most contemporary HF guidelines[3,7] but they will not be discussed in this review, which is focused on imaging.

Although echocardiography is the imaging technique most frequently used for a first evaluation of patients with HF, multimodality imaging is key to diagnose the etiology of HF and provides incremental prognostic value. Cardiac magnetic resonance (CMR) provides the unique characteristic of noninvasive myocardial tissue characterization, key aspect in differential diagnosis of cardiomyopathies.[8,9] Coronary computed tomography angiography is increasingly used to rule out the presence of ischemic heart disease (particularly in patients with low-to-intermediate pretest probability for coronary artery disease). In addition, nuclear cardiology techniques permit visualization of cellular metabolism and diagnosis of inflammatory causes of HF.

In this review article, an overview of the latest advances in multimodality imaging for diagnosis and risk stratification of patients with HF will be appraised. New diagnostic and prognostic imaging insights will be discussed.

PHENOTYPING HEART FAILURE

Currently international guidelines advocate the use of LVEF to phenotype HF into 3 categories: HF with reduced EF (LVEF ≤40%), HFmrEF (LVEF between 41% and 49%), and HFpEF (LVEF ≥50%).[3,7] The management and outcomes of the patients may vary significantly based on this LVEF-based classification. A recent meta-analysis including more than 120,000 patients with HF showed that patients with HFmrEF had better prognosis as compared with patients with HFrEF but similar prognosis as compared with patients with HFpEF.[10]

Furthermore, in the latest ACC/AHA guidelines, a new category of HF is highlighted: HF with improved EF including patients with HF and an initial LVEF less than 40% that improves to greater than 40% at follow-up.[7] Although improvement in LVEF is associated with better outcomes, it does not mean full myocardial recovery or normalization of LV function. In most patients, cardiac structural abnormalities, such as LV chamber dilatation and ventricular systolic and diastolic dysfunction, may persist, and most importantly, LVEF can decrease after withdrawal of pharmacological treatment. LVEF is an imperfect parameter of LV

performance because it only considers the change in volume of the LV and does not consider the effective stroke (forward) volume (eg, in patients with HF and severe mitral regurgitation). In addition, LVEF does not accurately reflect the structural changes that precede overt LV systolic dysfunction. The measurement of LV deformation by strain imaging has emerged as a powerful tool to accurately quantify myocardial mechanics, including longitudinal, circumferential, and radial deformation.[11] Strain is a dimensionless measurement of change in length between 2 points,[12] and LV GLS is defined as the change in the LV myocardial length of various LV myocardial segments between diastole and systole divided by the original end-diastolic length.[13] The measurement of LV GLS is more reproducible than the measurement of LVEF, and it is less influenced by loading conditions (**Fig. 1**).[11]

Impairment of LV GLS occurs earlier than impairment of LVEF. Several studies have demonstrated impaired LV GLS among asymptomatic patients with risk factors such as hypertension[14] and diabetes[15] and have normal LVEF. The underlying mechanism that explains the preservation of LVEF while LV GLS is impaired is the fact that LV circumferential shortening (determined by the midmyocardial layers) increases to compensate the impairment of LV GLS. The LV myocardium has specific disposition of the myocardial fibers: the subendocardial fibers are oriented as a right-handed helix while the subepicardial fibers show a left-handed helix orientation. The transition from the subendocardium to the subepicardium leads to the circumferentially oriented midwall fibers. Although the shortening of the subendocardial and subepicardial layers determine mainly the LV GLS, the shortening of the midmyocardial layers determines the circumferential strain. The LV subendocardium is often the first layer affected in a myocardial injury (ie, ischemia, pressure, or volume overload). Therefore, LV GLS impairs earlier than the circumferential strain, which tries to compensate and keep LV stroke volume and LVEF preserved. In individuals without HF and normal LVEF, LV GLS may be impaired in as much as 17% as shown in general population studies, probably reflecting the effects of aging on LV function,[16] and between 35% and 45% among individuals with diabetes.[17,18]

Among patients with HFpEF, the subanalysis of the Treatment Of Preserved Cardiac Function Heart Failure with an Aldosterone Antagonist trial showed that 66% of the patients had impaired LV GLS despite having an LVEF greater than 50% and 50% of the patients had an LV GLS less than 15.8%,[14] which is rather low considering

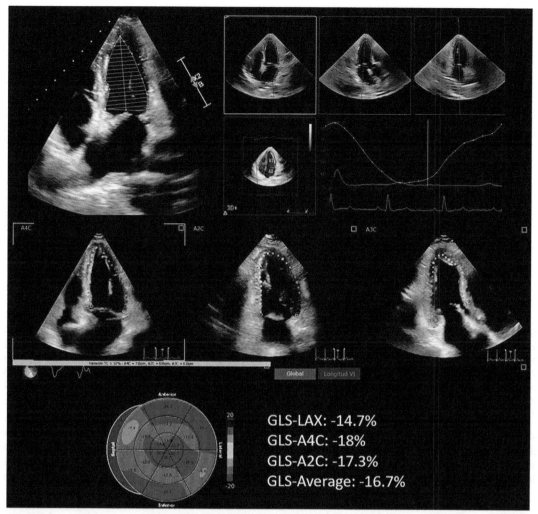

GLS-LAX: -14.7%
GLS-A4C: -18%
GLS-A2C: -17.3%
GLS-Average: -16.7%

Fig. 1. *Speckle tracking GLS of the left ventricle to detect subclinical left ventricular dysfunction.* Example of a 60-year-old woman receiving oncological therapy and showing impaired left ventricular GLS despite preserved LVEF measured with biplane 2D Simpson method (65%) and 3-dimensional echocardiography (58%). A2C, apical 2-chamber view; A4C, apical 4-chamber view; LAX, long-axis view.

that the lower limit of a normal value is 18%.[19] Importantly, each 1% decrease in LV GLS was associated with 14% increase in the risk of the primary composite outcome, HF hospitalization alone, and cardiovascular death alone.

Fig. 2 illustrates the underlying pathophysiological mechanisms explaining the discrepancy between LVEF and LV GLS. Any mechanical, ischemic, or metabolic myocardial injury leads to structural changes that consist of diffuse deposition of highly cross-linked collagen fibers and myocyte apoptosis and replacement fibrosis.[20] These structural derangements result in increased cardiomyocyte afterload and preload due to the collagen stiffening, impaired perfusion reserve due to perivascular fibrosis and capillary

rarefaction, and abnormal electrical conduction.[21] The extent and chronicity of these structural derangements will influence LV systolic and diastolic function that will be detected with LVEF and other parameters of diastolic function. However, LV GLS can reflect these structural changes at an earlier stage. LV GLS can be measured with echocardiography, CMR, and more recently ECG-gated computed tomography.[19–23] However, myocardial fibrosis is more frequently detected with CMR tissue characterization techniques. Particularly, diffuse reactive myocardial fibrosis is detected with T1 mapping, a quantitative method that tracks the recovery of the longitudinal magnetization of the tissue (**Fig. 3**). In native myocardium (without use of gadolinium), T1 relaxation time prolongs

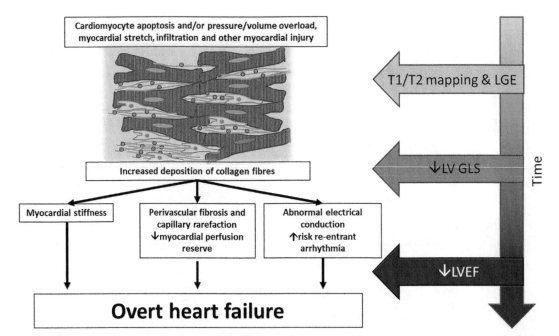

Fig. 2. *Time course of structural derangements of the myocardium and functional consequences evaluated with imaging techniques.* In response to myocardial injury and cardiomyocyte death, the extracellular matrix presents an increased deposition of collagen fibers and other cells that are profibrotic. At this time point, T1 and T2 mapping as well as LGE CMR can detect these early anatomical changes. The functional consequences can be detected with decreased left ventricular GLS while LVEF may remain normal. The initial deposition of collagen fibers leads to increased myocardial stiffness, perivascular fibrosis, and reduced myocardial perfusion and abnormal conduction increasing the risk of arrhythmias. Over time, these changes lead to overt HF when LVEF is reduced.

along with the amount of fibrosis of the myocardium, whereas the administration of gadolinium shortens the T1 relaxation time because the gadolinium accumulates in the increased interstitial space.[24] The extracellular volume (ECV) fraction can be calculated from the measurement of the T1 relaxation times pregadolinium and postgadolinium administration and has an excellent

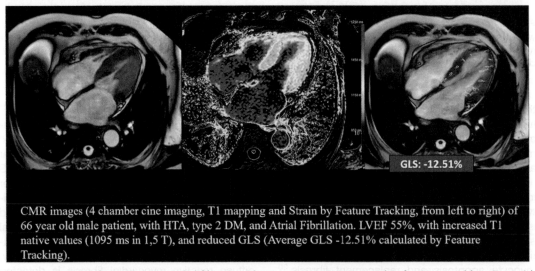

CMR images (4 chamber cine imaging, T1 mapping and Strain by Feature Tracking, from left to right) of 66 year old male patient, with HTA, type 2 DM, and Atrial Fibrillation. LVEF 55%, with increased T1 native values (1095 ms in 1,5 T), and reduced GLS (Average GLS -12.51% calculated by Feature Tracking).

Fig. 3. *Assessment of reactive myocardial fibrosis with T1 mapping CMR.* Example of a 66-year-old patient with arterial hypertension, diabetes mellitus, and atrial fibrillation. Left panel shows the cine image of the 4-chamber view. Note the dilated atria and thickened left ventricular myocardium. The central panel shows the T1 mapping sequence with an increased native T1 time of 1095 milliseconds. The panel on the right shows the assessment of GLS of the left ventricle with feature tracking, which results in an impaired value.

correlation with the ECV measured on histological samples. T1 mapping techniques have shown useful to identify and risk stratify patients with HFpEF.[24] In a prospective study of 112 individuals (62 with HFpEF, 22 with hypertension, and 28 healthy control subjects), an ECV fraction greater than 31.2% measured on CMR identified the patients with HFpEF with 100% sensitivity and 75% specificity.[25] In addition, together with LV GLS, ECV fraction was significantly associated with reduced exercise capacity. The hemodynamic consequences of increased ECV fraction were evaluated in an invasive study including 24 patients with HFpEF and 12 patients without HF who underwent pressure-volume loop analysis with conductance catheter.[24] Patients with more ECV fraction had stiffer LV and longer time of active LV relaxation, which was associated with hypertensive exercise response.

The structural changes that lead to LV dysfunction may cause as well alterations of the cardiac metabolism, which in turn may impair LV function. Phosphorus (31P)-magnetic resonance spectroscopy (MRS) offers a unique window into the assessment of high-energy phosphate metabolism. High-energy phosphates occupy a central position in cardiac metabolism, coupling oxygen, and substrate fuel delivery to the myocardium with contractile work. A reduction in the phosphocreatine (PCr)/adenosine triphosphate (ATP) ratio is an energetic sign common to numerous conditions that can predispose to HF.[26] Human cardiac 31P-MRS studies have documented reductions in myocardial PCr/ATP ratio in nonischemic cardiomyopathy,[27–29] HFpEF,[30] hypertrophic cardiomyopathy,[31,32] hypertensive hypertrophy with or without HF,[33,34] severe aortic stenosis with or without HF,[35–37] among others. A reduction in the PCr/ATP ratio predicts prognosis in nonischemic cardiomyopathy,[38] and may improve with trimetazidine in HF,[39] after aortic valve replacement,[37–40] after weight loss,[41] suggesting that reduced PCr/ATP ratio is not necessarily simply an age-related phenomenon, and that energetics may be central to disease pathogenesis.[26] Although this technique seems promising in the characterization of patients with HF, the feasibility in routine clinical practice is limited to centers with high expertise in this imaging technique.

CAUSE OF HEART FAILURE

Diagnosis of the underlying cause of HF is key to a personalized treatment. Ischemic heart disease is the most frequent cause of HF. A systematic review of multicenter HF treatment trials involving more than 40,000 patients during the past 30 years, coronary artery disease was the underlying cause of HF in nearly 65% of the patients.[42] This percentage is probably underestimated since the cause was not evaluated in a systemic manner in many trials (invasive coronary angiography was not systematically performed), and patients with a recent myocardial infarction, angina, or objective evidence of active ischemia were excluded.[42] The presence of significant coronary artery lesions in patients with HF is independently associated with a worse long-term outcome.[43] Therefore, an accurate diagnosis is important to implement secondary prevention measures to improve the outcomes. Noninvasive imaging tests, either anatomical or functional, are recommended in patients with an intermediate probability of coronary artery disease and an LVEF greater than 50%.[44] In patients with high probability of coronary artery disease, invasive coronary angiography is recommended and fractional flow reserve test is indicated to decide the need of revascularization. Recently, the 2021 ESC Practice Guidelines for the management of patients with HF upgraded the recommendation of performing a noninvasive computed tomography coronary angiography (CTCA) in patients with HF and an LVEF less than 50% while invasive coronary angiography is recommended in symptomatic patients who do not respond to treatment or have symptomatic ventricular arrhythmias and may be considered in patients with low-to-intermediate pretest probability of coronary artery disease.[3] CTCA provides information on coronary artery stenosis severity, as invasive coronary angiography does, and on characteristics of the arterial wall as well as coronary plaque features associated with an increased risk of ischemic events and plaque burden.[45] Furthermore, technological advances allow the assessment of the fractional flow reserve on computed tomography providing information on the hemodynamic consequences of the coronary stenosis.[46]

Nonischemic HF causes pose a greater diagnostic challenge than ischemic HF. Several causes of nonischemic HF have different pathophysiologic mechanisms that lead to LV dysfunction, and in addition, they may coincide with the presence of significant coronary artery disease. The 2021 ESC Practice Guidelines for the management of patients with HF proposed a new classification of the nonischemic cardiomyopathies[3]: valvular heart disease, hypertensive cardiomyopathy, infiltrative cardiomyopathy (sarcoid, hemochromatosis), familial/genetic cardiomyopathy, stress cardiomyopathy (Tako-tsubo), myocarditis (infectious, toxin or medication, immunological, hypersensitivity), and acquired diseases such as immuno-mediated diseases, cardiotoxicity, peripartum cardiomyopathy neuromuscular disorders, and heart rhythm–related and endocrine or metabolic diseases. These different causes lead to different patterns of LV (and right ventricular) remodeling and myocardial structural changes that are better appreciated with imaging techniques that provide information on the tissue characteristics. Accordingly, CMR with the use of late gadolinium contrast-enhanced (LGE) images and other quantitative parameters such as T1-mapping and T2-mapping, and T2*-mapping is the most frequently used technique to first approach the nonischemic causes (**Fig. 4**). The presence of subendocardial or transmural LGE in a territory that follows the supply of a coronary artery suggests the presence of significant coronary artery disease and previous myocardial infarction. In contrast, nonischemic causes show more focal, patchy or midwall, and subepicardial location of the LGE. For example, midwall septal LGE is characteristic of idiopathic dilated cardiomyopathy, whereas inferolateral basal midwall LGE is observed in Andersen-Fabry disease and focal epicardial LGE is characteristic of cardiac sarcoidosis. Patchy, multifocal distribution in the hypertrophied regions or the junctions between the right and left ventricle are observed in hypertrophic cardiomyopathy, whereas diffuse LGE pattern with poor differentiation between the myocardium and the blood pool is characteristic of cardiac amyloidosis.[47]

The presence of myocardial edema detected with T2-weighted CMR sequences suggests the diagnosis of acute myocarditis, and it is one of the Lake Louise Criteria. The combination of altered T2 mapping and subepicardial or midwall LGE in patients with symptoms and increased troponin has a median area under the curve to diagnose myocarditis of 0.90.[48] T2 mapping is also useful in infiltrative cardiomyopathies such as cardiac amyloidosis and Fabry disease. Myocardial iron deposition in primary hemochromatosis can lead to dilated cardiomyopathy that is characteristically detected with T2* mapping. In addition, the timing of chelation therapy and its effectiveness can be monitored with T2* mapping.

Positron emission tomography (PET) imaging with 18 F-fluorodeoxyglucose (FDG) is being increasingly recognized as a valuable tool in the detection and monitoring of inflammatory diseases. Increased FDG uptake is a hallmark of inflammation. Compared with CMR, FDG-PET represents a different and more direct visualization of myocarditis by quantifying the metabolic activity of inflammatory cell infiltrates. Several case reports and studies have highlighted the utility of hybrid FDG-PET/CMR in the assessment of inflammatory conditions of the heart such as viral myocarditis,[49,50] cardiac sarcoidosis,[51,52] and Loeffler endocarditis.[53] In patients with unexplained increased LV wall thickness, HFpEF, familial amyloid polyneuropathy, family history of amyloidosis, calcific aortic stenosis with low flow low gradient in the elderly, and a history of bilateral carpal tunnel syndrome, [99m]Technetium-bisphosphonate derivates scintigraphy facilitates the diagnosis of amyloid transthyretin (ATTR) cardiac amyloidosis.[54] The ratio of heart-to-contralateral lung uptake, heart-to-whole-body retention, and heart-to-bone ratio (visual grade) assessed at 1 and 3 hours after intravenous administration of bone-avid tracers are diagnostic parameters of cardiac amyloidosis on cardiac scintigraphy (**Fig. 5**). Perugini and colleagues demonstrated that a visual grade of 2 or greater on [99m]Technetium-3,3-diphosphono-1,2-propanodicarboxylic acid (^{99m}Tc-DPD) cardiac scintigraphy had a 100% sensitivity to identify ATTR cardiac amyloidosis and 100% specificity to differentiate from amyloid immunoglobulin light chain

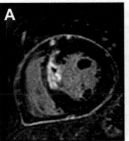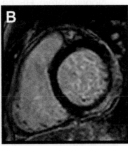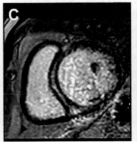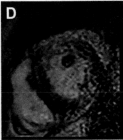

Fig. 4. *Late gadolinium-enhanced CMR to diagnose cause of HF.* Panel A shows an example of transmural myocardial infarction in the anterior interventricular septum. Subepicardial enhancement in the lateral and posterior walls of the left ventricle due to myocarditis is shown in panel B. Midwall fibrosis of the interventricular septum characteristic of idiopathic dilated cardiomyopathy is presented in panel C. Panel D shows concentric left ventricular hypertrophy with diffuse late gadolinium enhancement pattern and poor differentiation of the blood pool in a patient with cardiac transthyretin amyloidosis.

(AL) cardiac amyloidosis and controls.[55] It is important to emphasize that serum/urine immunofixation and serum free light chain assay excluding monoclonal process should be performed in all patients with suspected amyloidosis. In case of plasma cell dyscrasia, endomyocardial biopsy for histological diagnosis is still needed because 20% of patients with AL cardiac amyloidosis may show substantial uptake on cardiac scintigraphy.[56]

This extensive evidence highlights the key role of multimodality imaging in the etiologic diagnosis of nonischemic cardiomyopathies.

EXERCISE IMAGING

In many patients with HF symptoms, LV systolic function may be preserved and the hemodynamic evaluation at rest may not show the underlying pathophysiology of fluid accumulation in the systemic and pulmonary circulation. Congestion is the hallmark of HF and is influenced by various hemodynamic and nonhemodynamic factors. Exercise induces changes in loading conditions that may unmask LV diastolic dysfunction that leads to high left-sided filling pressures and transient pulmonary transcapillary transudation.[57] In patients with dyspnea and preserved LVEF, invasive hemodynamic exercise testing demonstrating a pulmonary capillary wedge pressure of 25 mm Hg or greater confirms the diagnosis of HFpEF.[58] Noninvasive imaging exercise testing has shown feasibility and accuracy in diagnosing HF. Exercise stress echocardiography allows the assessment of LV diastolic function, presence of LV wall motion abnormalities, and impairment of mitral and tricuspid regurgitation, which can cause lung congestion. In addition, during the same exercise stress echocardiography, lung ultrasound can be performed and the presence of B-lines, which have been associated with cardiovascular outcomes, can be detected.[59] The presence of an average E/e' ratio during exercise 15 mm Hg or greater and a peak tricuspid regurgitation velocity of greater than 3.4 m/s suggests the presence of HFpEF.[58] More recently, combined cardiopulmonary and exercise echocardiography stress testing has shown the value of additional echocardiographic parameters to predict peak oxygen consumption (VO_2). In 357 patients (113 at risk of developing HF and 244 with HFpEF or HFrEF), Pugliese and colleagues[60] showed that peak LV systolic annulus tissue velocity (S'), peak tricuspid annular plane systolic excursion/systolic pulmonary arterial pressure ratio (right ventricular-pulmonary arterial coupling) and left atrial compliance (measured as the ratio between left atrial reservoir strain and E/e' ratio) were independent predictors of VO_2. Using exercise-CMR, Backhaus and colleagues[61] demonstrated in 75 patients with echocardiographic signs of LV diastolic dysfunction and dyspnea on exertion that left atrial longitudinal strain during peak exercise was the most accurate parameter to detect HFpEF. Besides the structural changes that may underpin these functional abnormalities, it has been hypothesized that there may be an abnormal cardiac energetic state that impairs the active phase of the LV diastolic relaxation and leads to increased LV filling pressures and transient pulmonary congestion. This was demonstrated by Burrage and colleagues using phosphorous MRS and proton-density MRI sequence.[57] Across the spectrum of LV diastolic function (including 11

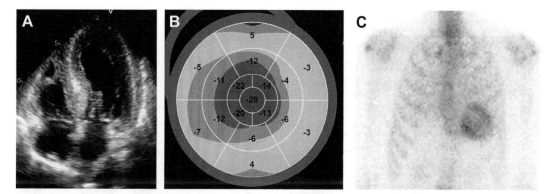

Fig. 5. *Diagnosis of transthyretin cardiac amyloidosis with scintigraphy.* Example of a 78-year-old patient with HF symptoms, bilateral tunnel carpal syndrome, and polyneuropathy symptoms in both legs. Panel A shows severe hypertrophy of the left and right ventricle. On speckle tracking analysis of left ventricular GLS, the typical apical cherry pattern with preserved shortening of the apical segments and impaired longitudinal strain of the mid and basal left ventricular segments can be observed (*B*). On ^{99m}Tc-DPD cardiac scintigraphy, the uptake of the tracer is clearly shown in panel C.

healthy controls, 9 patients with type 2 diabetes mellitus, 14 patients with HFpEF, and 9 patients with cardiac amyloidosis), there was a progressive reduction in PCr/ATP ratio (measure of cardiac energetic state) along with increasing E/e' ratio. In addition, impaired cardiac energetic state was associated with lower LV diastolic filling rates and diastolic reserve, more left and right atrial dilation and worse right ventricular contractile reserve during low-intensity exercise. Furthermore, transient pulmonary congestion was observed in patients with HFpEF and cardiac amyloidosis while it was not observed in healthy controls and patients with type 2 diabetes mellitus.

IMAGING FOR RISK STRATIFICATION OF HEART FAILURE

In recent trials including patients with HFrEF, advances in HF therapy have reduced significantly the proportion of deaths from a cardiac cause, whereas the proportion of noncardiovascular deaths has increased.[62] In patients with HFpEF, the mortality burden is also substantial and 50% to 70% of them are cardiovascular deaths, particularly driven by sudden cardiac death and HF death.[63] Compared with HFrEF, the proportions of cardiovascular deaths, sudden death and HF deaths are lower in HFpEF, whereas the proportion of noncardiovascular deaths in HFpEF exceeds that of HFrEF.[64] The majority of the studies evaluating the role of imaging for risk stratification of patients with HF have used as endpoint all-cause mortality. However, using cardiovascular death or HF-related death as endpoints may be more relevant. LVEF is the main parameter for risk stratification of HF regardless of the imaging technique used

to measure it. However, it has been shown that 30% of patients with ischemic HF receiving an implantable cardiac defibrillator as primary prevention based on the presence of HF symptoms and an LVEF less than 35% do not benefit during follow-up.[65] Characterization of the arrhythmogenic substrate considering specific myocardial scar tissue features, the heterogeneous electrical activation and the interaction with myocardial sympathetic innervation is key to identify the patients at higher risk of sudden cardiac death.

Several large studies have demonstrated the association between LGE extent (myocardial scar/fibrosis) on CMR and the occurrence of sudden cardiac death in ischemic and nonischemic cardiomyopathies.[66–68] In addition, specific features of myocardial scar have been associated with ventricular arrhythmias. For example, a ringlike pattern of scar (involving at least 3 contiguous segments in the same short-axis slice) has shown to be independently associated with the composite endpoint of all-cause death and cardiac arrest due to ventricular fibrillation or hemodynamically unstable ventricular tachyarrhythmia and appropriate implantable cardioverter defibrillator shock.[69] Furthermore, in patients with ischemic HF, the so-called periinfarct zone (border zone consisting of bundles of collagen intermingled with viable myocardial tissue) has been shown to have specific corridors where reentrant ventricular arrhythmias can occur.[70]

This anatomical substrate may become unstable with the alteration of the milieu due to ischemia, altered sympathetic innervation, or electrolytes for example. PET and single photon computed tomography can detect denervated, viable myocardium, which is associated with an

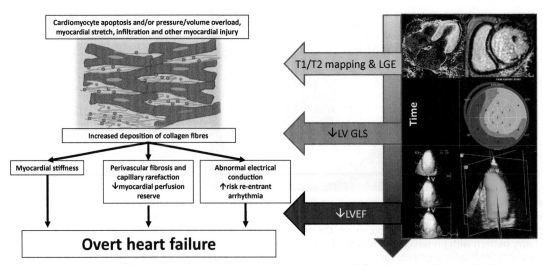

Fig. 6. Use of multimodality imaging to evaluate cardiac remodeling and function in patients with HF.

increased risk of ventricular arrhythmias. [123]Iodine-metaiodobenzylguanidine scintigraphy is the most frequently used imaging technique to detect cardiac sympathetic innervation. On planar imaging, a low heart-to-mediastinum uptake ratio of this radiotracer, indicating myocardial denervation, has been associated with an increased risk of ventricular arrhythmias and sudden cardiac death.[71]

This accumulating evidence showing the importance of characterizing the myocardial substrate for risk stratification in patients with HF has been underscore in recent ESC guidelines on the management of ventricular arrhythmias where a significant number of recommendations for the use of multimodality imaging have been included.[72]

SUMMARY

Multimodality imaging is key in the diagnosis of patients with HF symptoms (**Fig. 6**). Assessment of cardiac structure and function has increased in sophistication with the use of novel technologies such as strain imaging and assessment of cardiac energetics. Importantly, accurate diagnosis of cause of HF is key to provide a personalized treatment, and this requires the assessment of the myocardial tissue characteristics. Although endomyocardial biopsy remains the reference standard to define the cause, tissue characterization with noninvasive imaging modalities has become the first approach to diagnose the HF etiology.

CLINICS CARE POINTS

- HF is a heterogeneous clinical syndrome. Diagnosis of the underlying cause of HF by multimodality imaging is key to a personalized treatment.
- Phenotyping HF with LVEF is not sensitive enough to detect subclinical left ventricular systolic dysfunction in population at risk of HF (Stages A and B). Novel parameters of cardiac function, specially left ventricular GLS, have emerged as powerful tools to detect an early impairment of left ventricular function.
- Noninvasive exercise testing (with echocardiography and/or CMR imaging) may be helpful to unmask the underlying mechanisms of HF with preserved left ventricular ejection fraction (HFpEF). Myocardial energetic state may also play a role in the worsening of left ventricular diastolic function and transient lung congestion during exercise in patients with HFpEF.

DISCLOSURE

V. Delgado received speaker fees from Abbott Vascular, Edwards Lifesciences, GE Healthcare, Medtronic, Novartis, and Philips and consulting fees from Edwards Lifesciences and Novo Nordisk (heart failure).

REFERENCES

1. Savarese G, Lund LH. Global public health burden of heart failure. Card Fail Rev 2017;3:7–11.
2. Al-Mohammad A, Mant J, Laramee P, et al. Chronic Heart Failure Guideline Development Group. Diagnosis and management of adults with chronic heart failure: summary of updated NICE guidance. BMJ 2010;341:c4130.
3. McDonagh TA, Metra M, Adamo M, et al, ESC Scientific Document Group. 2021 ESC Guidelines for the diagnosis and treatment of acute and chronic heart failure Developed by the Task Force for the diagnosis and treatment of acute and chronic heart failure of the European Society of Cardiology (ESC). Eur Heart J 2021;42:3599–726.
4. Anker SD, Butler J, Filippatos G, et al. EMPEROR-Preserved Trial Investigators. Empagliflozin in Heart Failure with a Preserved Ejection Fraction. N Engl J Med 2021;385:1451–61.
5. Packer M, Butler J, Zannad F, et al. Effect of Empagliflozin on Worsening Heart Failure Events in Patients With Heart Failure and Preserved Ejection Fraction: EMPEROR-Preserved Trial. Circulation 2021;144:1284–94.
6. Vaduganathan M, Claggett BL, Inciardi RM, et al. Estimating the Benefits of Combination Medical Therapy in Heart Failure With Mildly Reduced and Preserved Ejection Fraction. Circulation 2022;145:1741–3.
7. Heidenreich PA, Bozkurt B, Aguilar D, et al. 2022 AHA/ACC/HFSA Guideline for the Management of Heart Failure. A Report of the American College of Cardiology/American Heart Association Joint Committee on Clinical Practice Guidelines. J Am Coll Cardiol 2022;79:1757–80.
8. Gonzalez JA, Kramer CM. Role of imaging techniques for diagnosis, prognosis and management of heart failure patients: cardiac magnetic resonance. Curr Heart Fail Rep 2015;12:276–83.
9. Messroghli DR, Moon JC, Ferreira VM, et al. Clinical recommendations for cardiovascular magnetic resonance mapping of T1, T2, T2 and extracellular volume: a consensus statement by the Society for Cardiovascular Magnetic Resonance (SCMR) endorsed by the European Association for Cardiovascular Imaging (EACVI). J Cardiovasc Magn Reson 2017;19:75.
10. Raja DC, Samarawickrema I, Das S, et al. Long-term mortality in heart failure with mid-range ejection

fraction: systematic review and meta-analysis. ESC Heart Fail 2022;9(6):4088–99.

11. Nesbitt GC, Mankad S, Oh JK. Strain imaging in echocardiography: methods and clinical applications. Int J Cardiovasc Imaging 2009;25(Suppl 1): 9–22.

12. Marwick TH, Shah SJ, Thomas JD. Myocardial Strain in the Assessment of Patients With Heart Failure A Review. JAMA Cardiol 2019;4:287–94.

13. Kinno M, Nagpal P, Horgan S, et al. Comparison of Echocardiography, Cardiac Magnetic Resonance, and Computed Tomographic Imaging for the Evaluation of Left Ventricular Myocardial Function: Part 2 (Diastolic and Regional Assessment). Curr Cardiol Rep 2017;19:6.

14. Imbalzano E, Zito C, Carerj S, et al. Left ventricular function in hypertension: New insights by speckle tracking echocardiography. Echocardiography 2011;28:649–57.

15. Fang ZY, Leano R, Marwick TH. Relationship between longitudinal and radial contractility in subclinical diabetic heart disease. Clin Sci (London) 2004; 106:53–60.

16. Russo C, Jin Z, Elkind MS, et al. Prevalence and prognostic value of subclinical left ventricular systolic dysfunction by global longitudinal strain in a community-based cohort. Eur J Heart Fail 2014;16: 1301–9.

17. Ernande L, Bergerot C, Rietzschel ER, et al. Diastolic dysfunction in patients with type 2 diabetes mellitus: is it really the first marker of diabetic cardiomyopathy? J Am Soc Echocardiogr 2011;24:1268–75.

18. Holland DJ, Marwick TH, Haluska BA, et al. Subclinical LV dysfunction and 10-year outcomes in type 2 diabetes mellitus. Heart 2015;101:1061–6.

19. Abou R, van der Bijl P, Bax JJ, et al. Global longitudinal strain: clinical use and prognostic implications in contemporary practice. Heart 2020;106:1438–44.

20. González A, Schelbert EB, Díez J, et al. Myocardial Interstitial Fibrosis in Heart Failure: Biological and Translational Perspectives. J Am Coll Cardiol 2018; 71:1696–706.

21. Schelbert EB. Myocardial Scar and Fibrosis: The Ultimate Mediator of Outcomes? Heart Fail Clin 2019; 15:179–89.

22. Podlesnikar T, Delgado V, Bax JJ. Cardiovascular magnetic resonance imaging to assess myocardial fibrosis in valvular heart disease. Int J Cardiovasc Imaging 2018;34:97–112.

23. Hirasawa K, Singh GK, Kuneman JH, et al. Feature-tracking computed tomography left atrial strain and long-term survival after transcatheter aortic valve implantation. Eur Heart J Cardiovasc Imaging 2023; 24(3):327–35.

24. Gupta S, Ge Y, Singh A, et al. Multimodality Imaging Assessment of Myocardial Fibrosis. JACC Cardiovasc Imaging 2021;14:2457–69.

25. Mordi IR, Singh S, Rudd A, et al. Comprehensive Echocardiographic and Cardiac Magnetic Resonance Evaluation Differentiates Among Heart Failure With Preserved Ejection Fraction Patients, Hypertensive Patients, and Healthy Control Subjects. JACC CV Imaging 2018;11:577–85.

26. Peterzan MA, Lewis AJM, Neubauer S, et al. Non-invasive investigation of myocardial energetics in cardiac disease using 31P magnetic resonance spectroscopy. Cardiovasc Diagn Ther 2020;10: 625–35.

27. Neubauer S, Krahe T, Schindler R, et al. 31P magnetic resonance spectroscopy in dilated cardiomyopathy and coronary artery disease. Altered cardiac high-energy phosphate metabolism in heart failure. Circulation 1992;86:1810–8.

28. Hardy CJ, Weiss RG, Bottomley PA, et al. Altered myocardial high-energy phosphate metabolites in patients with dilated cardiomyopathy. Am Heart J 1991;122:795–801.

29. Neubauer S, Horn M, Pabst T, et al. Contributions of 31P-magnetic resonance spectroscopy to the understanding of dilated heart muscle disease. Eur Heart J 1995;16:115–8.

30. Mahmod M, Pal N, Rayner J, et al. The interplay between metabolic alterations, diastolic strain rate and exercise capacity in mild heart failure with preserved ejection fraction: A cardiovascular magnetic resonance study. J Cardiovasc Magn Reson 2018;20:88.

31. Crilley JG, Boehm EA, Blair E, et al. Hypertrophic cardiomyopathy due to sarcomeric gene mutations is characterized by impaired energy metabolism irrespective of the degree of hypertrophy. J Am Coll Cardiol 2003;41:1776–82.

32. Ashrafian H, Redwood C, Blair E, et al. Hypertrophic cardiomyopathy:a paradigm for myocardial energy depletion. Trends Genet 2003;19:263–8.

33. Lamb HJ, Beyerbacht HP, van der Laarse A, et al. Diastolic Dysfunction in Hypertensive Heart Disease Is Associated With Altered Myocardial Metabolism. Circulation 1999;99:2261–7.

34. Smith CS, Bottomley PA, Schulman SP, et al. Altered Creatine Kinase Adenosine Triphosphate Kinetics in Failing Hypertrophied Human Myocardium. Circulation 2006;114:1151–8.

35. Conway MA, Allis J, Ouwerkerk R, et al. Detection of low phosphocreatine to ATP ratio in failing hypertrophied human myocardium by 31P magnetic resonance spectroscopy. Lancet 1991;338:973–6.

36. Neubauer S, Horn M, Pabst T, et al. Cardiac high-energy phosphate metabolism in patients with aortic valve disease assessed by 31P-magnetic resonance spectroscopy. J Investig Med 1997;45: 453–62.

37. Mahmod M, Francis JM, Pal N, et al. Myocardial perfusion and oxygenation are impaired during stress in severe aortic stenosis and correlate with

impaired energetics and subclinical left ventricular dysfunction. J Cardiovasc Magn Reson 2014;16:29.

38. Neubauer S, Horn M, Cramer M, et al. Myocardial Phosphocreatine-to-ATP Ratio Is a Predictor of Mortality in Patients With Dilated Cardiomyopathy. Circulation 1997;96:2190–6.

39. Fragasso G, Perseghin G, De Cobelli F, et al. Effects of metabolic modulation by trimetazidine on left ventricular function and phosphocreatine/adenosine triphosphate ratio in patients with heart failure. Eur Heart J 2006;27:942–8.

40. Beyerbacht HP, Lamb HJ, van der Laarse A, et al. Aortic Valve Replacement in Patients with Aortic Valve Stenosis Improves Myocardial Metabolism and Diastolic Function. Radiology 2001;219:637–43.

41. Rider OJ, Francis JM, Tyler D, et al. Effects of weight loss on myocardial energetics and diastolic function in obesity. Int J Cardiovasc Imaging 2013;29:1043–50.

42. Gheorghiade M, Sopko G, De Luca L, et al. Navigating the Crossroads of Coronary Artery Disease and Heart Failure. Circulation 2006;114:1202–13.

43. Smith SC Jr, Blair SN, Bonow RO, et al. AHA/ACC Scientific Statement: AHA/ACC guidelines for preventing heart attack and death in patients with atherosclerotic cardiovascular disease: 2001 update: a statement for healthcare professionals from the American Heart Association and the American College of Cardiology. Circulation 2001;104:1577–9.

44. Knuuti J, Wijns W, Saraste A, et al, ESC Scientific Document Group. 2019 ESC Guidelines for the diagnosis and management of chronic coronary syndromes. Eur Heart J 2020;41:407–77.

45. Williams MC, Kwiecinski J, Doris M, et al. Low-Attenuation Noncalcified Plaque on Coronary Computed Tomography Angiography Predicts Myocardial Infarction: Results From the Multicenter SCOT-HEART Trial (Scottish Computed Tomography of the HEART). Circulation 2020;141:1452–62.

46. Nørgaard BL, Gaur S, Fairbairn TA, et al. Prognostic value of coronary computed tomography angiographic derived fractional flow reserve: a systematic review and meta-analysis. Heart 2022;108:194–202.

47. Mahrholdt H, Wagner A, Judd RM, et al. Delayed enhancement cardiovascular magnetic resonance assessment of nonischaemic cardiomyopathies. Eur Heart J 2005;26(15):1461–74.

48. Eichhorn C Greulich S, Bucciarelli-Ducci C, Sznitman R, et al. Multiparametric Cardiovascular Magnetic Resonance Approach in Diagnosing, Monitoring, and Prognostication of Myocarditis. JACC Cardiovasc Imaging 2022;15:1325–38.

49. Nensa F, Poeppel TD, Krings P, et al. Multiparametric assessment of myocarditis using simultaneous positron emission tomography/magnetic resonance imaging. Eur Heart J 2014;35:2173.

50. Olshausen GV, Hyafil F, Langwieser N, et al. Detection of acute inflammatory myocarditis in epstein barr virus infection using hybrid 18F-fluoro-deoxy-glucose–positron emission tomography/magnetic resonance imaging. Circulation 2014;130:925–6.

51. White JA, Rajchl M, Butler J, et al. Active cardiac sarcoidosis: first clinical experience of simultaneous positron emission tomography-magnetic resonance imaging for the diagnosis of cardiac disease. Circulation 2013;127:e639–41.

52. Nensa F, Tezgah E, Poeppel T, et al. Diagnosis and treatment response evaluation of cardiac sarcoidosis using positron emission tomography/magnetic resonance imaging. Eur Heart J 2015;36:550.

53. Langwieser N, von Olshausen G, Rischpler C, et al. Confirmation of diagnosis and graduation of inflammatory activity of Loeffler endocarditis by hybrid positron emission tomography/magnetic resonance imaging. Eur Heart J 2014;35:2496.

54. Dorbala S, Ando Y, Bokhari S, et al. ASNC/AHA/ASE/EANM/HFSA/ISA/SCMR/SNMMI Expert Consensus Recommendations for Multimodality Imaging in Cardiac Amyloidosis: Part 1 of 2-Evidence Base and Standardized Methods of Imaging. Circ Cardiovasc Imaging 2021;14:e000029.

55. Perugini E, Guidalotti PL, Salvi F, et al. Noninvasive etiologic diagnosis of cardiac amyloidosis using 99mTc-3,3-diphosphono-1,2-propanodicarboxylic acid scintigraphy. J Am Coll Cardiol 2005;46:1076–84.

56. Gillmore JD, Maurer MS, Falk RH, et al. Nonbiopsy Diagnosis of Cardiac Transthyretin Amyloidosis. Circulation 2016;133:2404–12.

57. Burrage MK, Hundertmark M, Valkovič L, et al. Energetic Basis for Exercise-Induced Pulmonary Congestion in Heart Failure With Preserved Ejection Fraction. Circulation 2021;144:1664–78.

58. Pieske B, Tschöpe C, de Boer RA, et al. How to diagnose heart failure with preserved ejection fraction: the HFA-PEFF diagnostic algorithm: a consensus recommendation from the Heart Failure Association (HFA) of the European Society of Cardiology (ESC). Eur Heart J 2019;40:3297–317.

59. Picano E, Scali MC, Ciampi Q, et al. Lung Ultrasound for the Cardiologist. JACC Cardiovasc Imaging 2018;11:1692–705.

60. Pugliese NR, De Biase N, Conte L, et al. Cardiac Reserve and Exercise Capacity: Insights from Combined Cardiopulmonary and Exercise Echocardiography Stress Testing. J Am Soc Echocardiogr 2021;34:38–50.

61. Backhaus SJ, Lange T, George EF, et al. Exercise Stress Real-Time Cardiac Magnetic Resonance Imaging for Noninvasive Characterization of Heart Failure With Preserved Ejection Fraction: The HFpEF-Stress Trial. Circulation 2021;143:1484–98.

62. Rush CJ, Campbell RT, Jhund PS, et al. Falling Cardiovascular Mortality in Heart Failure With Reduced Ejection Fraction and Implications for Clinical Trials. JACC Heart Fail 2015;3:603–14.

63. Vaduganathan M, Patel RB, Michel A, et al. Mode of Death in Heart Failure With Preserved Ejection Fraction. J Am Coll Cardiol 2017;69:556–69.

64. Chan MM, Lam CS. How do patients with heart failure with preserved ejection fraction die? Eur J Heart Fail 2013;15:604–13.

65. Moss AJ, Greenberg H, Case RB, et al. Multicenter Automatic Defibrillator Implantation Trial-II (MADIT-II) Research Group. Long-term clinical course of patients after termination of ventricular tachyarrhythmia by an implanted defibrillator. Circulation 2004;110: 3760–5.

66. Kuruvilla S, Adenaw N, Katwal AB, et al. Late gadolinium enhancement on cardiac magnetic resonance predicts adverse cardiovascular outcomes in nonischemic cardiomyopathy: a systematic review and meta-analysis. Circ Cardiovasc Imaging 2014;7: 250–8.

67. Klem I, Klein M, Khan M, et al. Relationship of LVEF and Myocardial Scar to Long-Term Mortality Risk and Mode of Death in Patients With Nonischemic Cardiomyopathy. Circulation 2021;143:1343–58.

68. Ganesan AN, Gunton J, Nucifora G, et al. Impact of Late Gadolinium Enhancement on mortality, sudden death and major adverse cardiovascular events in ischemic and nonischemic cardiomyopathy: A systematic review and meta-analysis. Int J Cardiol 2018;254:230–7.

69. Muser D, Nucifora G, Muser D, et al. Prognostic Value of Nonischemic Ringlike Left Ventricular Scar in Patients With Apparently Idiopathic Nonsustained Ventricular Arrhythmias. Circulation 2021;143: 1359–73.

70. Fernández-Armenta J, Berruezo A, Andreu D, et al. Three-dimensional architecture of scar and conducting channels based on high resolution ce-CMR: insights for ventricular tachycardia ablation. Circ Arrhythm Electrophysiol 2013;6:528–37.

71. Jacobson AF, Senior R, Cerqueira MD, et al, ADMIRE-HF Investigators. Myocardial iodine-123 meta-iodobenzylguanidine imaging and cardiac events in heart failure. Results of the prospective ADMIRE-HF (AdreView Myocardial Imaging for Risk Evaluation in Heart Failure) study. J Am Coll Cardiol 2010;55:2212–21.

72. Zeppenfeld K, Tfelt-Hansen J, de Riva M, et al, ESC Scientific Document Group. 2022 ESC Guidelines for the management of patients with ventricular arrhythmias and the prevention of sudden cardiac death. Eur Heart J 2022;43:3997–4126.

Imaging in Hypertrophic Cardiomyopathy: Beyond Risk Stratification

Zachariah Nealy, MD[a], Christopher Kramer, MD[a,b],*

KEYWORDS

- Hypertrophic cardiomyopathy • Imaging • CMR • Echocardiography

KEY POINTS

- The main imaging modalities for diagnosing and evaluating hypertrophic cardiomyopathy include echocardiography and magnetic resonance.
- Imaging can predict atrial fibrillation burden, etiology of functional limitation, and sudden cardiac death risk.
- Imaging parameters play key roles in determining appropriateness of therapies, such as mavacamten and septal reduction therapy.

INTRODUCTION

The multimodality imaging approach to evaluating hypertrophic cardiomyopathy (HCM) has evolved substantially in parallel to treatment.[1,2] The prevalence of HCM historically was understood to be approximately one in 500, but recent data including increased use of cardiac magnetic resonance (CMR) as well as genetic testing to be closer to one in 200.[3] Patients may present asymptomatically or with symptoms and signs of left ventricular outflow tract (LVOT) obstruction, progressive heart failure, or arrhythmias. HCM is diagnosed when left ventricular wall thickness $\geq$ 15 mm in one or more segments or thickness $\geq$ 13 mm in the presence of known HCM-related sarcomere mutation or first-degree relatives with the diagnosis.[1,2] Any of the cardiac imaging modalities including echocardiography, CMR, or computed tomography (CT) can perform this measurement. Once diagnosed, patients are evaluated for the presence of obstruction, late gadolinium enhancement (LGE), systolic and diastolic dysfunction, functional limitations, burden of atrial and ventricular arrhythmias, and family history.[1,2] Although risk stratification for implantable cardioverter-defibrillator (ICD) placement and prevention of sudden cardiac death (SCD) are an important part of this workup, the role of advanced imaging in the care of HCM has evolved to include diagnostic, therapeutic, and prognostic decisions for the patient and their family members. This review focuses on the developing role of multimodality imaging in treatment of HCM (**Fig. 1**).

Diagnostic and Monitoring Parameters

HCM is typically detected by echocardiography, but CMR is often used when echocardiographic findings are either inconclusive or limited by available windows. The initial echocardiographic evaluation should include evaluation of maximum left ventricle (LV) wall thickness, LV ejection fraction (LVEF), diastolic function, left atrial chamber size, presence of LV apical aneurysm, valvular function and presence of systolic anterior motion (SAM), and LVOT obstruction (LVOTO).[1] Maximum LV wall thickness is best measured in the parasternal short and long axis views during end-diastole while avoiding the left and right ventricular

[a] Cardiovascular Division, Department of Medicine, University of Virginia Health, Charlottesville, VA 22908, USA; [b] Department of Radiology and Medical Imaging, University of Virginia Health, Charlottesville, VA 22908, USA
* Corresponding author. Cardiovascular Division, Department of Medicine, University of Virginia Health, 1215 Lee Street, Box 800158, Charlottesville, VA 22908.
E-mail address: ckramer@virginia.edu

Heart Failure Clin 19 (2023) 419–428
https://doi.org/10.1016/j.hfc.2023.03.004
1551-7136/23/© 2023 Elsevier Inc. All rights reserved.

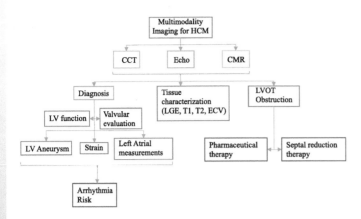

Fig. 1. The role of multimodality imaging in hypertrophic cardiomyopathy (HCM). CCT, cardiac computed tomography; CMR, cardiac magnetic resonance; LGE, late gadolinium enhancement; LVOT, left ventricular outflow tract.

trabeculations or papillary muscles when measuring septal thickness. There are multiple patterns of hypertrophy that vary by location along the septal, lateral, and apical segments. Owing to difficulties in image acquisition, foreshortening, difficulty with imaging windows, artifact or merely focal hypertrophy, there may be error in measuring maximum wall thickness.[4] In these cases, contrast-enhanced echocardiography and/or CMR may provide more accurate and reproducible measurements with less interobserver variability.[4,5] When evaluating wall thickness with CMR, measurements should be taken in the short axis with maximal measurement being used to evaluate for diagnostic criteria. In a study of 90 patients with confirmed HCM that underwent transthoracic echocardiography (TTE), transesophageal echocardiography (TEE) and CMR, in addition to CMR and TTE measurements correlating modestly, CMR more frequently delineated areas of maximal LV wall thickness other than the basal anteroseptum when compared with TTE and TEE.[6] Cine images of the four-chamber view can evaluate subtype morphology based on location and symmetry (or lack thereof) of wall thickness. The six main subtypes include localized basal septal hypertrophy, reverse curvature septal hypertrophy, apical HCM, concentric HCM, mid-cavity obstruction with apical aneurysm, and other that does not fit into the patterns of the other categories.[7]

Left Ventricular Function

LVEF should be measured using the biplane method of discs for echocardiography and volumetric coverage for CMR in instances where endocardial borders are poorly viewed on TTE. In HCM, LVEF is normal or hyperdynamic. Owing to LV hypertrophy, LV cavity size is often reduced resulting in low LV volumes. This can result in a low stroke volume and result in heart failure with preserved ejection fraction. LVEF less than 50% is defined as end stage among HCM patients and is associated with increased all-cause mortality, SCD, and need for cardiac transplantation or LVAD.[8] Measurement of diastolic dysfunction can be difficult as most individual echocardiographic Doppler measurements do not reflect diastolic dysfunction.[9] However, measurements that correlate with catheter-derived left atrial pressures include the ratio of early diastolic mitral inflow to mitral septal annular tissue velocity, left atrial enlargement, degree of hypertrophy, and transmitral Doppler ratio (E/A) of early diastolic ventricular filling velocities (E) to late diastolic ventricular filling velocities caused by atrial contraction (A)[10] **(Fig. 2)**.

Strain Imaging by Echocardiography and Cardiac Magnetic Resonance

Abnormal global longitudinal strain (GLS) and global circumferential strain (GCS) are early and sensitive signs of LV dysfunction. The ratio of endocardial strain to epicardial strain is an independent factor associated with LV maximal wall thickness.[11] By echocardiography, GLS has an incremental prognostic value for HCM and is associated with adverse outcomes including all-cause mortality, heart transplant, SCD, and later ICD implant.[12–14]

CMR-derived GCS also identifies differences between HCM and controls, but not between preclinical genotype positive–phenotype negative (GPPN) patients and controls. However, when the difference between epicardial and endocardial GCS was calculated, there was a significant difference between HCM patients, GPPN patients, and controls.[15] On CMR feature-tracking derived GLS, both 2-dimensional (2D) and 3-dimensional (3D) GLS were found to be independent predictors of adverse events among HCM patients and indicated that it could compound risk predicted by

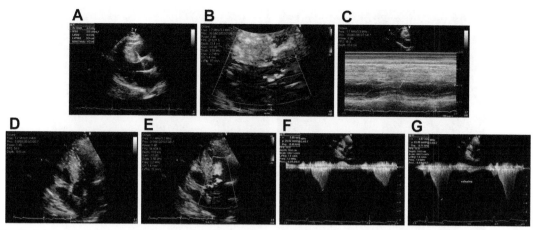

Fig. 2. Echocardiographic evaluation of left ventricular outflow tract (LVOT) for obstruction in hypertrophic cardiomyopathy. (*A*) Parasternal long-axis of the left ventricle with septum measuring 2.6 cm at end-diastole. (*B*) Parasternal long-axis with color Doppler during mid-systole showing turbulent flow in the LVOT consistent with flow acceleration. (*C*) M-mode across the mitral valve showing systolic anterior motion of the anterior mitral valve leaflet. (*D*) Apical five-chamber mid-systole without color Doppler. (*E*) Apical five-chamber mid-systole with color Doppler showing turbulent flow in the LVOT. (*F*) Continuous wave Doppler through the LVOT at rest showing a gradient measuring 29 mm Hg. (*G*) Continuous wave Doppler through the LVOT with Valsalva showing a gradient of 54 mm Hg.

the presence of LGE (discussed below) or reduced LVEF.[16] CMR feature tracking strain-derived GCS in the LV and LA were abnormal among patients with HCM despite normal LVEF.

Cardiac Magnetic Resonance: Tissue Characterization

LGE is based on the principle that scar and fibrosis cause prolonged myocardial contrast retention due to differential increased distribution of contrast in expanded extracellular space. LGE is a marker of replacement fibrosis. LGE measured at 4 or 5 standard deviations above the mean of signal in normal myocardium yielded the closest approximation with histopathological analysis of fibrosis in the myocardium removed during myectomy.[17] One meta-analysis found that the presence of and the extent of LGE on CMR correlate with an increased risk of SCD, all-cause mortality, cardiovascular mortality, and heart failure deaths.[18] The presence of LGE correlates with an increased risk of arrhythmia, adverse LV cavity remodeling, and predicts SCD but not when LVEF is diminished.[19] The absence of LGE also correlates with lower risk of SCD, arrhythmia, and development of symptoms.[20,21] T1 is sensitive to inflammation, edema, and fibrosis. T2 is sensitive to edema. Extracellular volume (ECV) is sensitive to fibrosis but less sensitive than T1. Fibrosis predicts adverse outcomes in HCM patient and can risk stratify to guide treatment. T1 and T2 combined have predicted genotype positivity in the absence of disease.[22–24]

Left Atrial Measurements

Left atrial chamber measurement correlates with prognosis, the risk of developing atrial fibrillation (AF), and diastolic dysfunction in patients with HCM.[14,25] CMR measured left atrial ejection fraction (LAEF) with LA remodeling correlates with the development of AF.[26] A study of 104 patients found that left atrial volume index linearly correlates with incidence of mitral regurgitation, degree of LV hypertrophy, adverse cardiovascular events, and diastolic dysfunction along with incidence of AF regardless of LVOTO status[27] (**Fig. 3**).

Valvular Evaluation

Valvular evaluation among patients with HCM predominantly focuses on the mitral valve for evaluation of regurgitation, SAM, and abnormalities of mitral apparatus including papillary muscle abnormalities and chordae. Screening usually occurs with echocardiography and is complimented by CMR. Mitral regurgitation is frequently recognized on echocardiography by evaluating apical and parasternal long axis views with color Doppler focused on the left atrium to evaluate the direction of the jets. The etiology is generally due to pathologic MV elongation and thickening, leaflet malcoaptation, and SAM, independent of the degree of hypertrophy.[28,29] Elongation is better detected by CMR.[30] Displacement of the papillary muscles can cause LVOTO or can compound LVOTO as the papillary hypertrophy will further reduce LVOT area. Mitral regurgitation worsens in a

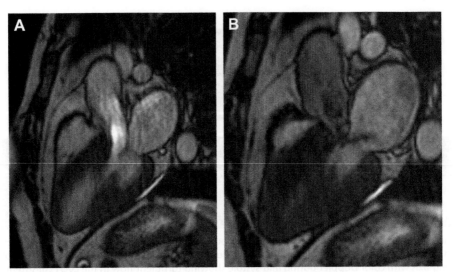

Fig. 3. Cardiac magnetic resonance of hypertrophic cardiomyopathy with LVOT obstruction. (*A, B*) Balanced steady-state free precession (B-SSFP) cine imaging of the three-chamber view at mid-systole and late systole, respectively. (*A*) Flow acceleration through the LVOT. (*B*) Chordal systolic anterior motion of the anterior leaflet of the mitral valve as well as significant eccentric mitral regurgitation.

proportional manner to severity of SAM and can be independent of or due to SAM. Mitral regurgitation due to SAM is normally directed laterally and posteriorly.[25] SAM is caused by the Venturi effect and drag force generated by LV contraction that causes LVOTO. Furthermore, hyperdynamic systolic function can worsen SAM. Other risk factors for SAM that can be evaluated on TTE and CMR include anterior mitral leaflet height greater than 1.5 cm, anterior: posterior leaflet length ratio less than 1.3, bulging subaortic septum, excess mitral leaflet tissue of either leaflet, and anterior and medial displacement of the papillary muscles.[31]

Left Ventricular Outflow Tract Obstruction

LVOTO is defined as resting or provocable peak gradient $\geq$ 30 mm Hg. Gradients $\geq$ 50 mm Hg can be the threshold for determination of myosin inhibitors or septal reduction therapies (SRTs) if patients have symptoms refractory to other medical therapy.[1,2] Obstruction will be apparent on echocardiography as turbulence on color Doppler. Gradients can be obtained by interrogating from the apex to the aortic valve with pulse wave Doppler to detect the presence of aliasing and confirm the level of the LVOTO. Continuous wave Doppler is used to measure the peak gradient.[2] The mechanisms of LVOTO include (1) reduced LVOT area from septal hypertrophy that anteriorly displaces the mitral valve leaflets and (2) hypertrophy and elongation of the mitral valve, apparatus, and papillary muscles that lead to anterior displacement. Both of these lead to abnormal

blood flow vectors causing SAM and leading to LVOTO, mitral regurgitation, and increased cavitary pressures.[1] Typically, this is dynamic and can be affected by increased contractility, reduced afterload and reduced preload, all of which will increase LVOT gradient.[1] Approximately 41% of patients have an LVOTO gradient $\geq$ 30 at rest and between 66% and 70% have a significant gradient with provocation.[32,33] LVOTO at rest is an independent predictor of symptoms of heart failure and death among patients with HCM.[34] Typical provocative maneuvers include Valsalva and/or exercise.[35–37] Eliciting LVOTO with provocative maneuvers is useful if no gradient at rest is detected. In one study of 50 symptomatic HCM patients without LVOTO receiving cardiac catheterization in the absence of provocative maneuvers, 40% were found to have been misclassified as less than severe LVOTO.[38] Exercise stress echocardiography can provoke a gradient among patients with latent obstruction.[39] This is more sensitive than Valsalva for eliciting these gradients after septal ablation.[40] Treadmill exercise seems to elicit greater maximum gradients when compared with supine bicycle.[41] When measuring LVOT gradient, it should be done at peak exercise to maximize the measured gradient (**Fig. 4**).

Left Ventricular Aneurysm

Left ventricular apical aneurysms are defined as thin-walled dyskinetic or akinetic segments located in the distal LV apex. These occur in a few percent of HCM patients who generally have

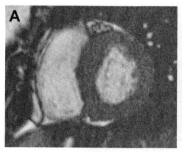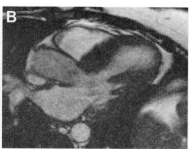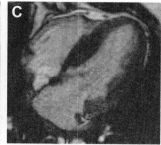

Fig. 4. Cardiac magnetic resonance of hypertrophic cardiomyopathy for measurement of wall thickness. (*A*) Short axis view of basal portion of ventricle measuring 17 mm. The three-chamber (*B*) and the four-chamber (*C*) can lead to overestimation or underestimation of wall thickness.

mid-cavity obstruction.[1,2] Aneurysm formation may be due to apical cavity pressure, ischemic thinning and scarring of the ape due to excess wall stress, or a combination of these factors.[42] Echocardiography can detect this and contrast echo and CT can also be helpful in detecting the aneurysm and possible apical thrombi as well.[43] CMR may be required for detection when there are obstructed echocardiographic apical views from near field clutter or apical foreshortening. Echocardiography can miss aneurysms in up to 43% of cases. These often require a high index of suspicion to detect.[44] This is particularly important as aneurysms are associated with an annual adverse event rate of 11% including ventricular arrhythmia and SCD[45] and are now an indication for an ICD based on most recent guidelines.[1]

Atrial Fibrillation Risk

Separate from risk stratification for SCD, imaging is useful for predicting and determining structural factors associated with developing AF-AFL among HCM patients. Among echocardiographic parameters, left atrial strain measured along with higher LA volumes and lower LAEF correlate with developing of paroxysmal AF among HCM patients.[46] In particular, low LA reservoir and conduit strain have the strongest relationship to the development of AF. ECV measurements were inversely related to LA conduit strain and directly to developing AF.[47]

CMR measurements similarly outlined associated structural changes. Out of HCM patients with and without AF, LGE in the LA was associated with the AF group. The study that noted this also found lower LAEF, higher LV LGE, and lower peak longitudinal LA strain in those with AF.[48] When measured by CMR, LA volume has a greater impact on predicting AF prevalence compared with left ventricular LGE.[49] Other CMR markers may also help to clarify the risk of AF[50] (**Figs. 5** and **6**).

Pharmacological Therapy

The role of multimodality imaging for therapy involves evaluating quantitative parameters, monitoring progression of disease and complications, and evaluating for adverse effects of pharmacologic therapy. Quantitative parameters obtained through echocardiography and CMR, such as LV wall thickness, LVOT gradient, LVEF, LV filling pressures (E/e'), and pulmonary artery (PA) pressures, may determine indication for and improvement with therapy.[1,2]

The first line of therapy for HCM with LVOTO is beta-blockers.[1] Beta-blockers reduce symptoms due to LVOTO, angina due to increased myocardial oxygen demand, and controls ventricular rate in AF if present.[1,51] Beta blockers are effective at modest reduction of LVOT gradients and improve latent LVOTO.[52,53] Beta blockers can reduce exercise capacity due to heart rate reduction while exercising despite the reduction in LVOT gradient.[54] Also, titration of beta blockers to an optimal LVOT gradient and reduction of symptoms may be beneficial for patients that are not candidates for invasive therapy or other forms of medical therapy.

Calcium channel blockers may be an acceptable alternative for those that are beta blocker intolerant for similar reasons as they improve myocardial oxygen consumption[55] and reduce LVOTO[56] and with less chronotropic incompetence.[57] Disopyramide is third-line therapy for obstructive HCM and similarly reduces LVOT gradient and improves symptoms but can lead to rapid conduction of AF.[58]

The most recent therapy for HCM, mavacamten, a cardiac myosin inhibitor, is indicated for those with LVOT gradient $\geq$ 50 mm Hg at rest or with provocation, EF greater than 55% and New York Heart Association (NYHA) class II to III symptoms. In addition to improvement of NYHA class symptoms and peak oxygen consumption (pVO$_2$), the intervention significantly reduced LVOT gradients in the EXPLORER-

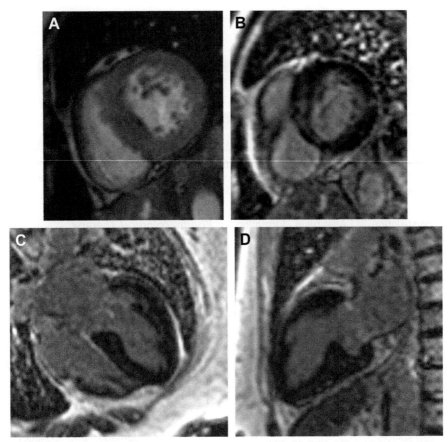

Fig. 5. (*A*) steady state free procession (SSFP) cine imaging of short axis measuring 17 mm consistent with hypertrophic cardiomyopathy, isolated basal septal subtype. (*B*) phase sensitive inversion recovery (PSIR) image in the short axis showing LGE in the mid-myocardium in mid-inferior, septal and lateral walls. (*C*) PSIR image in the four-chamber view showing LGE in the basal and mid-septal and lateral walls. (*D*) PSIR image in the two-chamber view showing LGE in the mid anterior and inferior walls.

HCM trial. In a CMR substudy, LV mass index and wall thickness were reduced as was left atrial volume index (LAVI). As expected with this negatively inotropic therapy, LVEF fell by 6.6%.[59] In the main EXPLORER cohort, there were nine patients noted by echocardiography to have a transient LVEF decrease to less than 50%.[60] Echocardiographic evaluation noted a reduction in E/e', LAVI, LVOT, and presence of SAM with therapy.[61] Regular echocardiography is required as part of the REMS

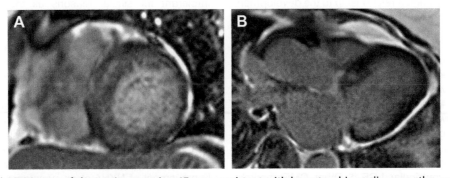

Fig. 6. (*A*) PSIR image of short axis measuring 17 mm consistent with hypertrophic cardiomyopathy, asymmetric basal septal subtype, showing mid wall LGE in the anteroseptum, inferoseptum, and inferior wall. (*B*) PSIR imaging of the three-chamber view showing LGE in the basal anteroseptal walls.

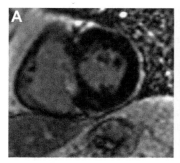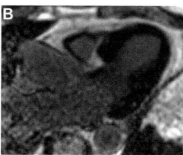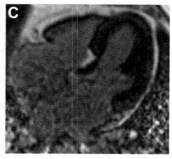

Fig. 7. CMR of patient with hypertrophic cardiomyopathy status post-septal alcohol ablation. (*A*) PSIR image of short axis view demonstrating dense scar involving the basal anteroseptum and inferoseptum. (*B*) PSIR image of three-chamber view showing dense basal scar along anteroseptum. (*C*) PSIR image of four-chamber view showing dense basal scar along inferoseptum.

program for instituting mavacamten therapy to ensure that the EF has not fallen below 50% with therapy.

Septal Reduction Therapy

SRTs are indicated in patients with symptomatic LVOTO despite optimal medical therapy. Both myectomy and septal ablation reduce LVOTO and improve NYHA functional class.[62] Myectomy improves survival when performed at high-volume centers.[63] Follow-up echocardiography is necessary to assure sustained reduction in LVOTO and formation of septal scars at 3 months and beyond.[64]

Intraoperative TEE for surgical myectomy helps plan extent of resection and actively evaluates SAM and LVOTO by color Doppler. It also evaluates the improvement of mitral regurgitation and assesses immediate results excluding surgical complications.[65] Intraoperative TEE directs the surgeons toward areas of continued obstruction with persistent gradients or continued mitral regurgitation.[66]

For alcohol septal ablation, TTE and TEE localize LAD septal perforators by intracoronary injection and monitor LVOT gradient reduction. Echocardiography, including contrast, improves procedural success of reducing LVOT gradient,[67] decreases intervention time, reduces size of infarct, and reduces chances of developing heart block as a complication.[1,2,68]

CMR also predicts adverse events for these procedures. Preoperative CMR finding of increased LA volume was associated with higher odds of developing postoperative AF following myectomy.[69] Preoperative LGE was strongly correlated with degree of small intramural coronary arteriole dysplasia found on histopathology after myectomy, amount of scar found on CMR postoperatively, and subsequent ventricular tachycardia (VT) frequency[70] (**Fig. 7**).

SUMMARY

Advanced imaging modalities are important in diagnosis, determination of treatment modalities, predicting treatment complications, and prognostication for patients with HCM. Multimodality approaches are essential for disease state monitoring and management of HCM patients.

CLINICS CARE POINTS

- Echocardiography is useful for screening, but in event of difficulty in diagnosis or characterization, contrast echocardiography and CMR provide higher accuracy of measurements.

- Left ventricular outflow tract (LVOT) obstruction can be latent in up to 70% of patients and should be evaluated using provocative measures for accuracy.

- Mavacamten is a new pharmacologic option for patients with LVOT gradient ≥ 50 mm Hg, EF greater than 55%, and NYHA class II–III symptoms but requires regular echocardiographic follow-up to avoid adverse events of LVEF decreasing to less than 50%.

DISCLOSURE

Z. Nealy has nothing to disclose. C. Kramer Research grants from BMS, Cytokinetics.

REFERENCES

1. Ommen SR, Mital S, Burke MA, et al. AHA/ACC Guideline for the Diagnosis and Treatment of Patients With Hypertrophic Cardiomyopathy. Circulation 2020;142(25). https://doi.org/10.1161/cir.00000 00000000937.

2. Elliott PM, Anastasakis A, Borger MA, et al. Authors/ Task Force m. 2014 ESC Guidelines on diagnosis and management of hypertrophic cardiomyopathy: The Task Force for the Diagnosis and Management of Hypertrophic Cardiomyopathy of the European Society of Cardiology (ESC). Eur Heart J 2014; 35(39):2733–79.

3. Semsarian C, Ingles J, Maron M, et al. New Perspectives on the Prevalence of Hypertrophic Cardiomyopathy. J Am Coll Cardiol 2015;65(12):1249–54.

4. Hindieh W, Weissler-Snir A, Hammer H, et al. Discrepant Measurements of Maximal Left Ventricular Wall Thickness Between Cardiac Magnetic Resonance Imaging and Echocardiography in Patients With Hypertrophic Cardiomyopathy. Circulation 2017;10(8).

5. Urbano-Moral JA, Gonzalez-Gonzalez AM, Maldonado G, et al. Contrast-Enhanced Echocardiographic Measurement of Left Ventricular Wall Thickness in Hypertrophic Cardiomyopathy: Comparison with Standard Echocardiography and Cardiac Magnetic Resonance. J Am Soc Echocardiogr 2020;33(9):1106–15.

6. Phelan D, Sperry BW, Thavendiranathan P, et al. Comparison of Ventricular Septal Measurements in Hypertrophic Cardiomyopathy Patients Who Underwent Surgical Myectomy Using Multimodality Imaging and Implications for Diagnosis and Management. Am J Cardiol 2017;119(10):1656–62.

7. Neubauer S, Kolm P, Ho C, et al. Distinct Subgroups in Hypertrophic Cardiomyopathy in the NHLBI HCM Registry. J Am Coll Cardiol 2019; 74(19):2333–45.

8. Marstrand P, Han L, Day SM, et al. Hypertrophic Cardiomyopathy With Left Ventricular Systolic Dysfunction. Circulation 2020;141(17):1371–83.

9. Rakowski H, Carasso S. Quantifying Diastolic Function in Hypertrophic Cardiomyopathy. Circulation 2007;116(23):2662–5.

10. Nistri S, Olivotto I, Betocchi S, et al. Prognostic significance of left atrial size in patients with hypertrophic cardiomyopathy (from the Italian Registry for Hypertrophic Cardiomyopathy). Am J Cardiol 2006; 98(7):960–5.

11. Tsugu T, Nagatomo Y, Dulgheru R, et al. Layer-specific longitudinal strain predicts left ventricular maximum wall thickness in patients with hypertrophic cardiomyopathy. Echocardiography 2021; 38(7):1149–56.

12. Li Y, Liu J, Cao Y, et al. Predictive values of multiple non-invasive markers for myocardial fibrosis in hypertrophic cardiomyopathy patients with preserved ejection fraction. Sci Rep 2021;11(1):4297.

13. Tower-Rader A, Mohananey D, To A, et al. Prognostic Value of Global Longitudinal Strain in Hypertrophic Cardiomyopathy. J Am Coll Cardiol Img 2019;12(10):1930–42.

14. Hiemstra YL, Debonnaire P, Bootsma M, et al. Global Longitudinal Strain and Left Atrial Volume Index Provide Incremental Prognostic Value in Patients With Hypertrophic Cardiomyopathy. Circulation 2017; 10(7).

15. Vigneault DM, Yang E, Jensen PJ, et al. Left Ventricular Strain Is Abnormal in Preclinical and Overt Hypertrophic Cardiomyopathy: Cardiac MR Feature Tracking. Radiology 2019;290(3):640–8.

16. Negri F, Muser D, Driussi M, et al. Prognostic role of global longitudinal strain by feature tracking in patients with hypertrophic cardiomyopathy: The STRAIN-HCM study. Int J Cardiol 2021;345:61–7.

17. Moravsky G, Ofek E, Rakowski H, et al. Myocardial fibrosis in hypertrophic cardiomyopathy: accurate reflection of histopathological findings by CMR. JACC 2013;6(5):587–96.

18. Weng Z, Yao J, Chan RH, et al. Prognostic Value of LGE-CMR in HCM: A Meta-Analysis. JACC 2016; 9(12):1392–402.

19. Ismail TF, Jabbour A, Gulati A, et al. Role of late gadolinium enhancement cardiovascular magnetic resonance in the risk stratification of hypertrophic cardiomyopathy. Heart 2014;100:1851–8.

20. Chan RH, Maron BJ, Olivotto I, et al. Prognostic Value of Quantitative Contrast-Enhanced Cardiovascular Magnetic Resonance for the Evaluation of Sudden Death Risk in Patients With Hypertrophic Cardiomyopathy. Circulation 2014;130(6): 484–95.

21. Rubinshtein R, Glockner JF, Ommen SR, et al. Characteristics and Clinical Significance of Late Gadolinium Enhancement by Contrast-Enhanced Magnetic Resonance Imaging in Patients With Hypertrophic Cardiomyopathy. Circulation 2010;3(1):51–8.

22. Ho CY, Abbasi SA, Neilan TG, et al. T1 Measurements Identify Extracellular Volume Expansion in Hypertrophic Cardiomyopathy Sarcomere Mutation Carriers With and Without Left Ventricular Hypertrophy. Circulation 2013;6(3):415–22.

23. Rao S, Tseng SY, Pednekar A, et al. Myocardial Parametric Mapping by Cardiac Magnetic Resonance Imaging in Pediatric Cardiology and Congenital Heart Disease. Circulation 2022;15(1). https://doi.org/10.1161/circimaging.120.012242.

24. Menghoum N, Vos JL, Pouleur AC, et al. How to evaluate cardiomyopathies by cardiovascular magnetic resonance parametric mapping and late gadolinium enhancement. Eur Heart J Card Img 2022; 23(5):587–9.

25. Geske JB, Sorajja P, Nishimura RA, et al. Evaluation of Left Ventricular Filling Pressures by Doppler Echocardiography in Patients with Hypertrophic Cardiomyopathy. Circulation 2007;116(23):2702–8.

26. Maron BJ, Haas TS, Maron MS, et al. Left atrial remodeling in hypertrophic cardiomyopathy and susceptibility markers for atrial fibrillation identified by

cardiovascular magnetic resonance. Am J Cardiol 2014;113(8):1394–400.

27. Yang H, Woo A, Monakier D, et al. Enlarged left atrial volume in hypertrophic cardiomyopathy: a marker for disease severity. J Am Soc Echocardiogr 2005; 18(10):1074–82.

28. Maron MS, Olivotto I, Harrigan C, et al. Mitral valve abnormalities identified by cardiovascular magnetic resonance represent a primary phenotypic expression of hypertrophic cardiomyopathy. Circulation 2011;124:40–7.

29. Woo A, Jedrzkiewicz S. The Mitral Valve in Hypertrophic Cardiomyopathy. Circulation 2011;124(1): 9–12.

30. Maron MS, Olivotto I, Harrigan C, et al. Mitral Valve Abnormalities Identified by Cardiovascular Magnetic Resonance Represent a Primary Phenotypic Expression of Hypertrophic Cardiomyopathy. Circulation 2011;124(1):40–7.

31. Ibrahim M, Rao C, Ashrafian H, et al. Modern management of systolic anterior motion of the mitral valve. Eur J Cardio Thorac Surg 2012;41(6):1260–70.

32. Shah JS, Esteban MT, Thaman R, et al. Prevalence of exercise-induced left ventricular outflow tract obstruction in symptomatic patients with non-obstructive hypertrophic cardiomyopathy. Heart 2008;94:1288–94.

33. Maron MS, Olivotto I, Zenovich AG, et al. Hypertrophic Cardiomyopathy Is Predominantly a Disease of Left Ventricular Outflow Tract Obstruction. Circulation 2006;114(21):2232–9.

34. Maron MS, Olivotto I, Betocchi S, et al. Effect of Left Ventricular Outflow Tract Obstruction on Clinical Outcome in Hypertrophic Cardiomyopathy. N Engl J Med 2003;348(4):295–303.

35. Joshi S, Patel UK, Yao SS, et al. Standing and Exercise Doppler Echocardiography in Obstructive Hypertrophic Cardiomyopathy: The Range of Gradients with Upright Activity. J Am Soc Echocardiogr 2011;24(1):75–82.

36. Marwick TH, Nakatani S, Haluska B, et al. Provocation of latent left ventricular outflow tract gradients with amyl nitrite and exercise in hypertrophic cardiomyopathy. Am J Cardiol 1995;75(12):805–9.

37. Feiner E, Arabadjian M, Winson G, et al. Post-Prandial Upright Exercise Echocardiography in Hypertrophic Cardiomyopathy. J Am Coll Cardiol 2013; 61(24):2487–8.

38. Geske J, Sorajja P, Ommen S, et al. Variability of Left Ventricular Outflow Tract Gradient During Cardiac Catheterization in Patients With Hypertrophic Cardiomyopathy. J Am Coll Cardiol Intv 2011;4(6):704–9.

39. Ayoub C, Geske JB, Larsen CM, et al. Comparison of Valsalva Maneuver, Amyl Nitrite, and Exercise Echocardiography to Demonstrate Latent Left Ventricular Outflow Obstruction in Hypertrophic Cardiomyopathy. Am J Cardiol 2017;120(12):2265–71.

40. Jensen MK, Havndrup O, Pecini R, et al. Comparison of Valsalva manoeuvre and exercise in echocardiographic evaluation of left ventricular outflow tract obstruction in hypertrophic cardiomyopathy. Eur J Echocardiogr 2010;11(9):763–9.

41. Reant P, Dufour M, Peyrou J, et al. Upright treadmill vs. semi-supine bicycle exercise echocardiography to provoke obstruction in symptomatic hypertrophic cardiomyopathy: a pilot study. Eur J Cardio Thorac Surg 2018;19(1):31–8.

42. Binder J, Attenhofer Jost CH, Klarich KW, et al. Apical hypertrophic cardiomyopathy: prevalence and correlates of apical outpouching. J Am Soc Echocardiogr 2011;24(7):775–81.

43. Cardim N, Galderisi M, Edvardsen T, et al. Role of multimodality cardiac imaging in the management of patients with hypertrophic cardiomyopathy: an expert consensus of the European Association of Cardiovascular Imaging Endorsed by the Saudi Heart Association. Eur J Cardio Thorac Surg 2015;16(3):280.

44. Maron MS, Finley JJ, Bos JM, et al. Prevalence, Clinical Significance, and Natural History of Left Ventricular Apical Aneurysms in Hypertrophic Cardiomyopathy. Circulation 2008;118(15):1541–9.

45. To A, Dhillon A, Desai M, et al. Cardiac Magnetic Resonance in Hypertrophic Cardiomyopathy. J Am Coll Cardiol Img 2011;4(10):1123–37.

46. Vasquez N, Ostrander BT, Lu DY, et al. Low Left Atrial Strain Is Associated With Adverse Outcomes in Hypertrophic Cardiomyopathy Patients. J Am Soc Echocardiogr 2019;32(5):593–603.

47. Tayal B, Malahfji M, Buergler JM, et al. Hemodynamic determinants of left atrial strain in patients with hypertrophic cardiomyopathy: A combined echocardiography and CMR study. PLoS One 2021;16(2):e0245934.

48. Sivalokanathan S, Zghaib T, Greenland GV, et al. Hypertrophic Cardiomyopathy Patients With Paroxysmal Atrial Fibrillation Have a High Burden of Left Atrial Fibrosis by Cardiac Magnetic Resonance Imaging. JACC 2019;5(3):364–75.

49. Papavassiliu T, Germans T, Flüchter S, et al. CMR findings in patients with hypertrophic cardiomyopathy and atrial fibrillation. J Cardiovasc Magn Reson 2009;11(1):34.

50. Kramer C, DiMarco J, Kolm P, et al. Predictors of Major Atrial Fibrillation Endpoints in the National Heart, Lung, and Blood Institute HCMR. J Am Coll Cardiol EP 2021;7(11):1376–86.

51. Cohen LS, Braunwald E. Amelioration of Angina Pectoris in Idiopathic Hypertrophic Subaortic Stenosis with Beta-Adrenergic Blockade. Circulation 1967;35(5):847–51.

52. Stenson RE, Flamm MD Jr, Harrison DC, et al. Hypertrophic subaortic stenosis. Clinical and hemodynamic effects of long-term propranolol therapy. Am J Cardiol 1973;31(6):763–73.

53. Nistri S, Olivotto I, Maron MS, et al. β Blockers for prevention of exercise-induced left ventricular outflow tract obstruction in patients with hypertrophic cardiomyopathy. Am J Cardiol 2012;110(5):715–9.

54. Gilligan D, Chan W, Joshi J, et al. A double-blind, placebo-controlled crossover trial of nadolol and verapamil in mild and moderately symptomatic hypertrophic cardiomyopathy. J Am Coll Cardiol 1993;21(7):1672–9.

55. Wilmshurst PT, Thompson DS, Juul SM, et al. Effects of verapamil on haemodynamic function and myocardial metabolism in patients with hypertrophic cardiomyopathy. Heart 1986;56:544–53.

56. Rosing DR, Kent KM, Borer JS, et al. Verapamil therapy: a new approach to the pharmacologic treatment of hypertrophic cardiomyopathy. I. Hemodynamic effects. Circulation 1979;60(6):1201–7.

57. Ammirati E, Contri R, Coppini R, et al. Pharmacological treatment of hypertrophic cardiomyopathy: current practice and novel perspectives. Eur J Heart Fail 2016;18:1106–18.

58. Sherrid M, Barac I, McKenna W, et al. Multicenter study of the efficacy and safety of disopyramide in obstructive hypertrophic cardiomyopathy. J Am Coll Cardiol 2005;45(8):1251–8.

59. Olivotto I, Oreziak A, Barriales-Villa R, et al. EXPLORER-HCM study investigators. Mavacamten for treatment of symptomatic obstructive hypertrophic cardiomyopathy (EXPLORER-HCM): a randomised, double-blind, placebo-controlled, phase 3 trial. Lancet 2020;396(10253):759–69 [Erratum in: Lancet. 2020 Sep 12;396(10253):758].

60. Saberi S, Cardim N, Yamani M, et al. Mavacamten Favorably Impacts Cardiac Structure in Obstructive Hypertrophic Cardiomyopathy. Circulation 2021; 143(6):606–8.

61. Hegde S, Lester S, Solomon S, et al. Effect of Mavacamten on Echocardiographic Features in Symptomatic Patients With Obstructive Hypertrophic Cardiomyopathy. J Am Coll Cardiol 2021;78(25): 2518–32.

62. Sorajja P, Valeti U, Nishimura RA, et al. Outcome of Alcohol Septal Ablation for Obstructive Hypertrophic Cardiomyopathy. Circulation 2008;118(2):131–9.

63. Ommen S, Maron B, Olivotto I, et al. Long-Term Effects of Surgical Septal Myectomy on Survival in Patients With Obstructive Hypertrophic Cardiomyopathy. J Am Coll Cardiol 2005;46(3):470–6.

64. Liebregts M, Vriesendorp P, Mahmoodi B, et al. A Systematic Review and Meta-Analysis of Long-Term Outcomes After Septal Reduction Therapy in Patients With Hypertrophic Cardiomyopathy. J Am Coll Cardiol HF 2015;3(11):896–905.

65. Grigg LE, Wigle ED, Williams WG, et al. Transesophageal Doppler echocardiography in obstructive hypertrophic cardiomyopathy: clarification of pathophysiology and importance in intraoperative decision making. J Am Coll Cardiol 1992;20(1): 42–52.

66. Marwick TH, Stewart WJ, Lever HM, et al. Benefits of intraoperative echocardiography in the surgical management of hypertrophic cardiomyopathy. J Am Coll Cardiol 1992;20(5):1066–72.

67. Faber L, Ziemssen P, Seggewiss H. Targeting percutaneous transluminal septal ablation for hypertrophic obstructive cardiomyopathy by intraprocedural echocardiographic monitoring. J Am Soc Echocardiogr 2000;13(12):1074–9.

68. Faber L, Seggewiss H, Ziemssen P, et al. Intraprocedural myocardial contrast echocardiography as a routine procedure in percutaneous transluminal septal myocardial ablation: Detection of threatening myocardial necrosis distant from the septal target area. Cathet Cardiovasc Intervent 1999;47:462–6.

69. Tang B, Song Y, Cheng S, et al. In-Hospital Postoperative Atrial Fibrillation Indicates a Poorer Clinical Outcome after Myectomy for Obstructive Hypertrophic Cardiomyopathy. Ann Thorac Cardiovasc Surg 2020;26(1):22–9.

70. Kwon DH, Smedira NG, Rodriguez ER, et al. Cardiac magnetic resonance detection of myocardial scarring in hypertrophic cardiomyopathy: correlation with histopathology and prevalence of ventricular tachycardia. J Am Coll Cardiol 2009;54(3): 242–9.

Arrhythmogenic Cardiomyopathy
Evolving Diagnostic Criteria and Insight from Cardiac Magnetic Resonance Imaging

Sohaib Ahmad Basharat, MD[a], Ingrid Hsiung, MD[b], Jalaj Garg, MD, FESC[a],
Amro Alsaid, MD, FSCMR[b],*

KEYWORDS

- Arrhythmogenic cardiomyopathy (ACM) • Genotyping
- Arrhythmogenic right ventricular cardiomyopathy (ARVC) • Dilated cardiomyopathy
- Hereditary cardiomyopathy • Cardiac sarcoidosis • Sudden cardiac death (SCD)
- Cardiac magnetic resonance imaging (CMR, MRI)

KEY POINTS

- Arrhythmogenic cardiomyopathy (ACM) is a term that encompasses a wide spectrum of hereditary conditions with variable phenotypic expression as well as a variety of nonhereditary conditions that predispose patients to arrhythmias.
- The revised 2010 Task Force criteria improved the specificity for detection of the right-dominant (arrhythmogenic right ventricular cardiomyopathy/dysplasia) phenotype but did not address phenotypes with isolated left-sided or left-dominant disease. The 2020 Padua criteria included left-dominant phenotypes and incorporated the diagnostic value of cardiac MRI in detecting structural cardiac abnormalities on late Gadolinium-enhanced imaging.
- Cardiac MRI (CMR) plays an essential role in the diagnosis of various forms of ACM, detecting high-risk features that warrant interventions, and is an extremely useful tool for serial follow-up in asymptomatic subclinical gene carriers.
- Genetic testing has a paramount importance in caring for patients with ACM and their families. A multidisciplinary individualized approach integrating the patient's clinical presentation, imaging, and genetic counseling should be implemented to guide clinical decision-making.
- Potential future care directions include incorporating CMR-based quantitative parameters and tissue characterization (T1, T2, and extracellular volume) to develop risk stratification calculators that aid in clinical decision-making and management of affected and subclinical individuals.

INTRODUCTION

Arrhythmogenic right ventricular dysplasia (ARVD) is a heritable disorder characterized by loss of ventricular myocardium and fibrofatty tissue replacement, resulting in structural cardiac abnormalities and ventricular arrhythmias. It was originally identified and reported in 1982 by Marcus and colleagues in a series of 24 patients with right ventricular (RV) arrhythmias.[1] The label evolved overtime to arrhythmogenic RV cardiomyopathy (ARVC) and arrhythmogenic left ventricular

[a] Division of Cardiology, Loma Linda University Medical Center, 11234 Anderson Street, MC2426, Loma Linda, CA 92354, USA; [b] Department of Cardiology, Baylor Scott & White The Heart Hospital, 1100 Allied Drive, Plano, TX 75093, USA
* Corresponding author.
E-mail address: amro.alsaid@bswhealth.org
Twitter: @drjalajgarg (J.G.); @AmroAlsaid (A.A.)

Heart Failure Clin 19 (2023) 429–444
https://doi.org/10.1016/j.hfc.2023.03.006
1551-7136/23/© 2023 Elsevier Inc. All rights reserved.

Abbreviations	
ACM	Arrhythmogenic Cardiomyopathy
CMR	Cardiac magnetic resonance
ARVD	Arrhythmogenic right ventricular dysplasia
ARVC	Arrhythmogenic right ventricular cardiomyopathy
DCM	Dilated Cardiomyopathy

cardiomyopathy (ALVC) or left-dominant arrhythmogenic cardiomyopathy (LDAC) to highlight phenotypes with biventricular or predominantly LV involvement.[2]

Most of the initial research interest was directed toward the originally described RV-dominant ARVD/ARVC. The original diagnostic criteria as well as management guidelines were also focused on the same entity.[3] However, the term arrhythmogenic cardiomyopathy (ACM) has been proposed to encompass a wide spectrum of arrhythmia-related cardiac conditions including a variety of hereditary, systemic, infectious, and inflammatory disorders (**Fig. 1**). This evolving understanding was reflected in the 2019 heart rhythm society (HRS) expert statement, where ACM was defined as "*arrhythmogenic heart muscle disorder not explained by ischemic, hypertensive, or valvular heart disease.*"[4]

Arrhythmogenic Cardiomyopathy

ACM thus refers to a heterogenous and variable phenotypic expression of overlapping disorders that carry an increased risk of cardiac arrhythmias and sudden cardiac death (SCD). This designation includes hereditary disorders such as classic ARVC, ALVC/LDAC, desmoplakin (DSP) cardiomyopathy, arrhythmic forms of dilated cardiomyopathy (DCM), arrhythmic mitral valve prolapse (MVP)/mitral annular disjunction (MAD), titin-associated cardiomyopathy, LMNA/C-related dilated cardiomyopathy, and phospholamban cardiomyopathy; varied channelopathies; as well as infiltrative systemic disorders such as sarcoidosis, amyloidosis; and infectious conditions such as Chagas disease.[4,5]

Histopathology and Genetics

Desmosomal proteins play a key role in myocardial cell-to-cell adhesion, and mutations in these genes lead to loss of sarcomeric connections and myocyte apoptosis. Desmosomes are also part of the Wnt-β-catenin signaling pathway that suppresses the expression of adipogenic and fibrogenic genes. Mutations of the desmosomal genes leads to malfunction of this pathway, resulting in a switch from myogenesis to fibrogenesis resulting in the fibrofatty replacement of myocardium.

The fibrofatty replacement was originally described in ARVC to involve the RV free wall, progressing from epicardium to endocardium, and resulting in wall thinning and aneurysm formation. Anatomically, a pathologic "triangle of dysplasia" was described between the inflow tract (subtricuspid), outflow tract (infundibulum), and the apex of the right ventricle where the disease was frequently noted to be localized. More recently a biventricular triangle of dysplasia has been described where the LV posterolateral wall replaces the RV apex and is reportedly the more common area of pathology particularly in ACM cases early in the disease course.[6]

In addition to fibro-fatty replacement of the cardiac myocytes, mutant desmosomal proteins lead to malignant ventricular arrhythmias by gap-junction remodeling, which leads to alterations in the sodium current resulting in depolarization and repolarization abnormalities. This pathophysiology explains the similar arrhythmic mechanisms between ACM and Brugada syndrome given their common origin from the connexome.[7]

The pathophysiological role of the desmosomal gene mutation was first described by Dr. Nikos Protonotarios on the Greek island of Naxos in a syndromic variant of the disease, the *Naxos disease*. It is an autosomal recessive variant of ARVC with a familial penetrance of ~90% and results in triad of palmoplantar keratosis and wooly hair in addition to cardiac manifestations. The responsible gene for this disease was identified on chromosome 17 and is responsible for

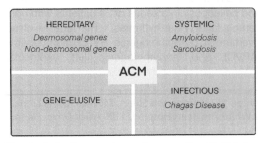

Fig. 1. Arrhythmogenic cardiomyopathy (ACM) is a broad term encompassing multiple disease entities associated with increased risk of malignant arrhythmias and sudden cardiac death.

producing Plakoglobin, which is a cytoplasmic component of the desmosomes/adherens junctions that are located within the intercalated discs and anchor the sarcomeres together.[8]

This discovery was a milestone in the understanding of ARVC/D and led to foundational research in identifying mutations of other desmosomal proteins related to ACM. Mutations in genes encoding desmosomal proteins such as DSP, plakophilin 2 (PKP2), desmoglein 2, and desmocollin 2 have been shown to cause the autosomal dominant forms of ACM.

Later, genes encoding nondesmosomal proteins were also implicated in pathogenesis of ACM. These proteins include ion channels and cytoskeletal components of the intercalated discs. Examples of such nondesmosomal proteins include LMNA, desmin, filamin C, and phospholamban.[9]

Moreover, some ACM cases were noted to have a hereditary pattern with no discernible gene mutation (*gene-elusive*). In one large study of patients with ACM, 37% had no identifiable gene mutation in the desmosomal, PLN, or TMEM43 genes. Among these gene-elusive cases, only one-fifth had evidence of familial disease.[10] These gene-elusive cases raise the question if they have a primarily monogenic disease or whether they represent an oligogenic form of ACM with unknown, low-penetrant genetic variants.

In patients who meet the Task Force diagnostic criteria, successful genotyping is noted in approximately 50% of the patients.[11] Further challenge also lies in differentiating causative mutations from nonpathogenic variants and gene polymorphisms.

CLINICAL PRESENTATION

Most cases of ACM (especially hereditary forms) manifest between second and fifth decades of life and can have variable initial cardiac presentation ranging from palpitations to SCD. In various series of patients with ACM, symptoms at presentation have been described as follows: palpitations (27%–67%), syncope (26%–32%), SCD (10%–26%), atypical chest pain (27%), and heart failure/dyspnea (11%).[12,13]

Even within a certain ACM subgroup, clinical presentations tend to be heterogeneous. Four different disease phases have been described[14]:

1. Concealed phase: this preclinical phase of the disease is characterized by asymptomatic individuals who nevertheless may be at an increased risk of malignant ventricular arrhythmias and SCD. This phase tends to have minimal to no detectable structural abnormalities by conventional imaging but may show subtle evidence of replacement fibrosis or subclinical diffuse interstitial fibrosis on cardiac MRI.[15]

2. Electrical phase: individuals in this phase might present with palpitations, syncope, or aborted cardiac arrest and may have premature ventricular contractions, nonsustained ventricular tachycardia, or sustained ventricular tachycardia. Structural ventricular abnormalities may be detected on various imaging modalities.

3. Progressive phase: this phase is characterized by worsening RV, LV, or biventricular structural abnormalities that are often combined with ventricular arrhythmias.

4. End-stage disease: patients might develop significant ventricular failure with or without ventricular arrhythmias. In this phase, ACM can be misdiagnosed as idiopathic nonischemic cardiomyopathy.

These phases of the disease are merely descriptive in nature and a particular patient does not necessarily go through all these phases sequentially. For example, although most patients might be first diagnosed in the electrical phase, others present with the "end-stage" phase of advanced heart failure without having any prior events.

SCD is the most feared outcome of ACM, and early diagnosis of the disease is critical for prevention. Although ARVC pattern has traditionally been thought of as the most common variant in patients presenting with SCD, more recent autopsy studies suggest that LV involvement might actually be predominant in patients with SCD.[16]

ACM can exhibit quiescent phases alternating with intermittent bursts of increased morbidity. These so-called *hot phases* can occasionally present as myocarditis-like episodes characterized by chest pain, ST-segment and T-wave changes on electrocardiogram (EKG) with elevated troponin levels. Inflammatory infiltrates (mainly T lymphocytes) have been observed in these cases masquerading as acute myocarditis. Alternatively, it has been theorized that inflammation and myocarditis might be triggers for phenotypic expression of ACM in asymptomatic gene carriers.[17,18]

In a systematic review, these *"hot phase"* episodes were suspected to be exercise induced in nearly 50% of the cases. Two-thirds of the patients who experienced these episodes were noted to have ALVC pattern of ACM. Most of these individuals were initially diagnosed as having acute myocarditis as can be expected given similar clinical presentations. On subsequent genetic testing, DSP was noted to be the most common gene (69%) in patients presenting with hot phase of the disease as opposed to the PKP2 gene mutation, which is most frequent in general ACM population.[19]

CLINICAL DIAGNOSIS

In 1994, an international task force (ITF) proposed guidelines to diagnose ARVC based on criteria from 6 categories (**Table 1**). Various findings in these categories were classified as major and minor criteria, and the diagnosis required the presence of either 2 major criteria, 1 major plus 2 minor, or 4 minor criteria from different categories.[3]

Subsequently, the task force criteria was revised in 2010 to improve specificity by including objective criteria for RV dysfunction and dilatation as well as the addition of cardiac MRI (CMR) for morphologic RV assessment (see **Table 1**).[20] However, despite the 2010 update, the sensitivity for diagnosis remained low, given inclusion of only RV predominant forms in the diagnostic criteria. In 2020, the Padua criteria was introduced, which included LV morphologic criteria

for the first time hence recognizing LV predominant or biventricular forms of the ACM (**Table 2**). The Padua criteria also highlighted the value of CMR and included tissue characterization by late-Gadolinium enhancement (LGE) for detection of fibrofatty myocardial replacement of either the right or left ventricle.[21]

ROLE OF IMAGING IN DIAGNOSIS AND MANAGEMENT OF ARRHYTHMOGENIC CARDIOMYOPATHY

As noted earlier, the diagnostic criteria are greatly reliant on cardiac imaging to detect morphofunctional and structural cardiac abnormalities. Although echocardiography is most often the initial imaging in the workup for ACM cases, it lacks sensitivity and specificity in comparison to CMR. Echo images can be affected by patient positioning and body habitus and thus focal chamber dilatation, microaneurysms, or dyskinesis might be missed. In addition, traditional echocardiographic functional assessment is susceptible to

---

Table 1
A comparison between the original task force criteria (1994) and the revised task force criteria (2010) for diagnosis of ARVC

Original Task Force Criteria (1994)	Revised Task Force Criteria (2010)
Global or regional dysfunction and structural alterations	
Subjective criteria for RV dilatation, dysfunction, aneurysms	Expanded objective criteria for RV dilatation and dysfunction based on either 2D echo, MRI, or RV angiography
Tissue characterization of wall	
Fibrofatty replacement of myocardium on endomyocardial biopsy	Objective criteria for loss of myocytes with or without fibrofatty replacement on endomyocardial biopsy
Repolarization abnormalities	
Inverted T waves in right precordial leads (only minor criteria)	Inverted T waves in right precordial leads (as major criteria) and other precordial leads (minor criteria)
Depolarization abnormalities	
Epsilon waves as major and SAECG late potentials as minor criteria	Original criteria plus an expanded list of depolarization abnormalities as minor criteria
Arrhythmias	
LBBB-VT and PVCs (only minor criteria)	LBBB-VT as major criteria. RVOT-VT and PVCs as minor criteria
Family history	
Family member with autopsy-confirmed ARVC, family member with suspected ARVC-related SCD, and family history of clinically diagnosed ARVC	Original criteria and addition of positive pathogenic mutation in the patient undergoing evaluation

Abbreviations: LBBB, left bundle branch block; RVOT, right ventricular outflow tract; SAECG, signal-averaged electrocardiography; 2D, two-dimensional.
Data from Refs.[3,20]

Table 2
Key points of the 2020 Padua criteria for diagnosis of arrhythmogenic cardiomyopathy

Padua Criteria for Diagnosis of ACM	
RV Criteria (Modified from 2010 TFC)	**LV Criteria (New Addition)**
Morphofunctional ventricular abnormalities	
RV dilatation, dysfunction, or dyskinesia/bulging by echo, CMR, or angiography (major and minor criteria)	Global LV dysfunction, dilatation, or hypokinesia/akinesia by echo, CMR, or angiography (only minor criteria)
Structural myocardial abnormalities	
LGE criteria on CE-CMR and fibrofatty replacement on EMB (major criteria)	LGE criteria on CE-CMR (major criteria)
Repolarization abnormalities	
Inverted T waves in right precordial leads as major criteria, other T-wave inversions as minor criteria	Inverted T waves in left precordial leads as minor criteria only
Depolarization abnormalities	
Epsilon wave and terminal activation duration (minor criteria)	Low QRS voltage in limb leads (minor criteria)
Ventricular arrhythmias	
Frequent PVCs, NSVT, or VT with LBBB morphology as major criteria and with LBBB-RVOT pattern as minor criteria	Frequent PVCs, NSVT, or VT with RBBB morphology as minor criteria
Family history/genetics	
Major and minor criteria for family history of ACM	
Major criteria for pathogenic ACM mutation in patient undergoing evaluation	

Adapted from Corrado D, Perazzolo Marra M, Zorzi A, et al. Diagnosis of arrhythmogenic cardiomyopathy: The Padua criteria. *Int J Cardiol.* 2020;319:106-114.

interreader variability and is prone to error due to geometric assumption of the morphology of cardiac chambers. Moreover, echocardiography lacks the ability to detect subtle cardiac structural abnormalities and signs of fibrofatty replacement. All these factors make echocardiogram a less dependable imaging modality for detecting early subclinical phenotypes or for long-term surveillance of patients with ACM.[22]

Cardiac MRI in arrhythmogenic cardiomyopathy

CMR provides accurate quantitative assessment of the cardiac function and chamber size without geometric assumptions (**Fig. 2**). It also offers the ability to obtain high-resolution images in standard and nonstandard imaging planes even in patients with challenging body habitus that is ideal for initial diagnosis and serial follow-up.[22]

Advances in CMR imaging sequences and development of parametric mapping allow generation of pixel-based, color-coded myocardial maps to detect various subtle abnormalities. These abnormalities include (1) subclinical interstitial fibrosis (using native precontrast T1, postcontrast T1 and extracellular volume [ECV] mapping), (2) myocardial edema/active inflammation (using T2 mapping), (3) fatty infiltration (using fat suppression sequences), and (4) replacement fibrosis (using late post-Gadolinium enhancement [LGE]) (**Fig. 3**). In particular, the degree of LGE has been shown as an independent predictor of ventricular arrhythmias.[23]

CMR also aids in differentiation of ACM from less common conditions such as congenital pericardial agenesis. CMR tissue strain analysis is promising to provide diagnostic and prognostic information in the future. Strain imaging can differentiate ACM from other conditions such as RV outflow tract-ventricular tachycardia and Brugada syndrome. CMR has also shown utility in differentiating ACM from athlete's heart by measuring strain rate of the midventricular RV free wall.[24] The multiple roles of CMR in diagnosis of variant ACM phenotypes are shown in **Fig. 4**. These roles are briefly described later.

In *DCM*, the pattern of LGE can provide clues to the cause. For example, patients with ischemic DCM may have subendocardial or transmural LGE, whereas those with nonischemic DCM may have patchy distribution of LGE with subepicardial or

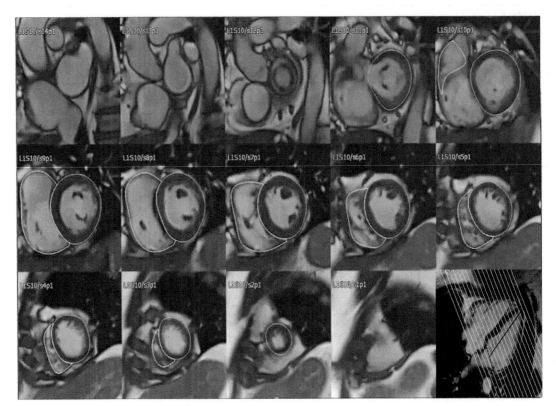

Fig. 2. CMR assessment of cardiac chambers and function is performed using multiple sequential short-axis cine slices covering the entire heart.

midwall location (**Fig. 5**). A study by Halliday and colleagues found that among patients with DCM and LV ejection fraction greater than or equal to 40%, presence of midwall LGE on CMR is associated with increased risk of SCD. These patients may benefit from implantable cardioverter defibrillator (ICD) implantation irrespective of LVEF.[25]

In *cardiac sarcoidosis (CS)*, CMR role extends beyond establishing the diagnosis of CS, as it allows detection of phenotypes with high risk for SCD who may benefit from ICD implantation. A recent study by Athwal and colleagues found that *pathology-frequent* LGE (reported as lesions located in LV subepicardial, LV multifocal, septal, or RV free wall) was associated with higher incidence of arrhythmic and heart failure events regardless of LVEF and LV LGE. Identification of such phenotypes can optimize decision-making regarding ICD implantation in the future.[26] CMR can also assess presence or absence of myocardial edema (**Fig. 6**), which can help in CS management, as patients with no edema and persistent atypical enhancement show little response to steroid therapy.[27]

In *cardiac amyloidosis*, CMR shows characteristic global subendocardial LGE with abnormal myocardial and blood-pool late-gadolinium kinetics noted due to cardiac amyloid deposits; this was also correlated with overall amyloid burden and LV mass that serves as a morphologic marker of amyloid load.[28] These characteristic findings can help distinguish cardiac amyloidosis from phenocopies (eg, hypertrophic cardiomyopathy, hypertensive or valvular cardiac disease, glycogen storage disorders, and Anderson-Fabry disease) (**Fig. 7**). No LGE-based criteria have been validated yet for prophylactic ICD implantation in cardiac amyloidosis but LGE is increasingly seen as proportional to the degree of amyloidosis and might have potential to predict malignant arrhythmias. The presence of expanded myocardial interstitial space can be evaluated by T1 and ECV mapping; this can serve as a surrogate for interstitial fibrosis[29] and can in future help with the diagnosis as well as assessment of interval changes after therapy.[30]

In *arrhythmic MVP/mitral annular disjunction (MAD)*, renewed interest has emerged in using cardiac imaging to subclassify patient with MVP who are at an increased risk for ventricular arrhythmia (VA) and SCD. LGE detected on CMR correlates with histopathological fibrosis, and certain identifiable patterns, for example, focal papillary muscle fibrosis or inferobasal scar in patients with MVP, have been linked to increased risk of VT/SCD[5]

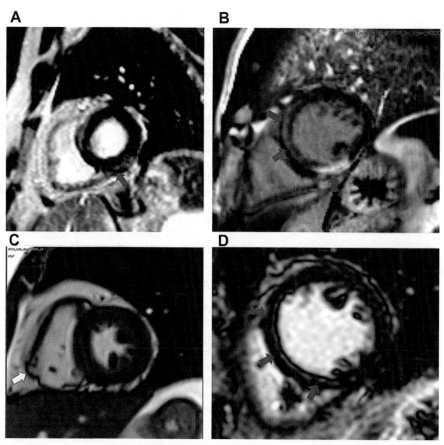

Fig. 3. CMR findings in 4 individual ACM gene carriers. Red arrows denote atypical LGE in the left ventricle. (*A*) Atypical midwall LGE in the basal to midinferior segment of a 59-year-old DSP-variant carrier. (*B*) Marked atypical LGE in a 57-year-old male DSP variant carrier subsequently diagnosed with ARVC. (*C*) Cine image showing a microaneurysm in the inferobasal RV segment in a 32-year-old DSG2-variant carrier (*white arrow*). (*D*) Atypical midwall septal LGE in a 34-year-old PKP2 variant carrier.

(**Fig. 8**). There is also a growing interest in exploring the role of surgical repair for MVP/MAD to reduce VA and risk of SCD irrespective of degree of mitral regurgitation, and CMR can be valuable in guiding the clinical decision-making by identifying the degree of MVP, assessing the extent of leaflet involvement, quantifying degree of mitral regurgitation and cardiac remodeling as well as identification and quantification of interstitial fibrosis and replacement fibrosis. It has also been noted that the pattern and degree of LV fibrosis differs between MVP- and non–MVP-related mitral regurgitation, supporting the hypothesis that MVP-related VA has a unique pathophysiology beyond cardiac remodeling due to chronic volume overload.[5]

RISK STRATIFICATION AND MANAGEMENT OF ARRHYTHMOGENIC CARDIOMYOPATHY

Current therapeutic options for patients with ACM include lifestyle modifications (including exercise restriction), β-blockers, antiarrhythmic drugs, ICD placement, catheter ablation, and heart transplantation. Importantly, a timely establishment of the correct diagnosis in cases of arrhythmic systemic or infectious subset of patients allows for initiation of appropriate disease-specific agents such as antiparasitic therapy in Chagas disease, immunosuppressive therapy in CS and emerging therapeutic agents in cardiac amyloidosis.

Implantable Cardioverter Defibrillator Placement

A main focus of intervention ACM revolves around identifying patients who are at a high risk of malignant arrhythmias in whom instituting early ICD implantation is critical in preventing sustained ventricular arrhythmias and SCD; this, however, remains challenging, and the risk of life-threatening arrhythmias has to be weighed against treatment-associated morbidities (eg, procedural

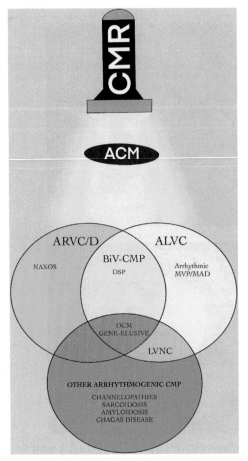

Fig. 4. Role of CMR in evaluation and differentiation of ACM. ACM, arrhythmogenic cardiomyopathy; ALVC, arrhythmogenic left ventricular cardiomyopathy; ARVC/D, arrhythmogenic right ventricular cardiomyopathy/dysplasia; BiV-CMP, biventricular cardiomyopathy; CMP, cardiomyopathy; CMR, cardiac MRI; DCM, dilated cardiomyopathy; DSP, desmoplakin.

complications of device implantation, physical and psychological burden of inappropriate shocks after device implantation).

Multiple risk stratification tools have been devised to estimate risk of malignant ventricular arrhythmias or SCD in patients with ACM. These tools include the 2015 International Task Force algorithm, which incorporates multiple factors including initial presentation, frequency and type of arrhythmia, EKG characteristics, and imaging characteristics. The ITF algorithm stratifies patients into low, intermediate, or high risk of SCD and provides recommendation for ICD implantation.[31] Although the ITF algorithm has a good overall ability to predict ventricular arrhythmias, it does not adequately distinguish this risk between those implanted for a class I or class IIa indication. This limitation is most likely to affect young patients

with ACM who tend to disproportionately experience malignant ventricular arrhythmia early in their disease course. More recently, a risk calculator has been developed to calculate a 5-year risk of ventricular arrhythmias and SCD in patients with confirmed diagnosis of ARVC. When compared with the ITF criteria, the newer ARVC risk calculator is reported to have a similar protection from SCD while reducing the total number of ICD implants by 20.3%.[32]

In contrast to these ARVC-focused risk calculators, the 2019 HRS expert consensus statement clinical decision-making algorithm considered the broader ACM term and incorporated other hereditary forms of ACM that are not just limited to ARVC/D when providing recommendations for ICD implantation (**Fig. 9**).[4]

ABLATION THERAPY

Ablation in patients with ACM does not modify the underlying arrhythmogenic substrate or progression of the disease but is rather aimed at improving quality of life by controlling symptoms and preventing repeated ICD therapies. Unlike VT related to ischemic cardiomyopathy, where the substrate tends to correlate with coronary distribution, involves the endocardium, and can be mapped and accessed from the endocardial surface, catheter ablation in ACM remains challenging, as the location of substrate tends to be less predictable, frequently requiring an epicardial or a combined endocardial and epicardial approach.[4]

During ablation procedures, voltage mapping is considered the "gold standard" for detection of myocardial scar "border zone" or myocardial channels. However, voltage mapping has few limitations due to a single endocardial (or epicardial) voltage measurement representing a poor surrogate for a complex midmyocardial scar distribution, limited spatial resolution of the electroanatomic maps, long mapping times, and falsely low-voltage measurements due to imperfect catheter contact.[33] Improved MRI, on the other hand, can accurately delineate myocardial scar (even in most patients with implantable ICD). Electroanatomic voltage mapping by 3-dimensional MRI scar reconstructions is showing promise to facilitate VT ablations.[34]

ROLE OF GENETIC TESTING IN DIAGNOSIS AND SCREENING

Genetic testing for patients plays an essential role in the care for suspected patients with ACM. Most of the hereditary ACM forms have autosomal

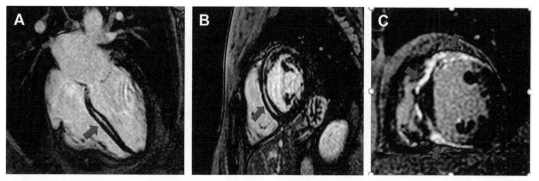

Fig. 5. Findings in 2 individuals with diagnosis of nonischemic dilated cardiomyopathy (DCM). Red arrows denote atypical LGE. Long-axis (*A*) and short axis (*B*) cardiac views revealing a characteristic nonischemic midwall linear LGE pattern in a 42-year-old patient with palpitations and mild left ventricular dysfunction subsequently diagnosed with TTN gene mutation. (*C*) Extensive nonischemic LGE involving the anterior septal and inferior walls in a patient with recurrent VT found to have LMNA cardiomyopathy.

dominant transmission although some autosomal recessive forms also exist. Because many subtypes of hereditary ACM show incomplete penetrance and phenotypic variability, this often results in underdiagnosis. Moreover, ACM can carry an indolent course in gene carriers with initial presentation often being SCD. These challenges highlight the importance of cascade genetic screening for family members of identified probands with the aim to identify the disease in

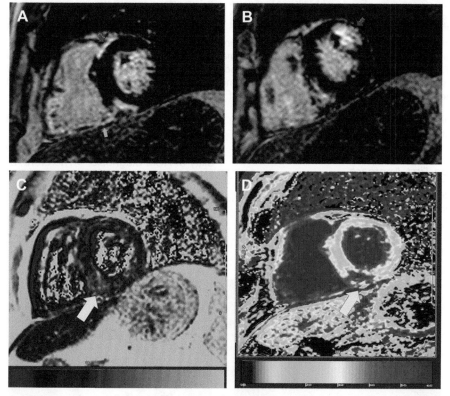

Fig. 6. Short-axis images in a patient initially suspected to have right ventricular outflow tract (RVOT) VT. CMR revealed multifocal nonischemic enhancement patterns. (*A*) Subepicardial LGE involving the anterior and inferoseptal segments (*red arrows*) and RV wall enhancement (*blue arrow*). (*B*) Atypical midwall LGE involving the anterolateral segment (*red arrow*). (*C, D*) T2 parametric mapping revealed elevated T2 decay time (*white arrow* in [*C*]) and increased extracellular volume ECV (*white arrow* in [*D*]) suggesting active inflammation. Patient was confirmed to have cardiac sarcoidosis and responded to immunosuppressive therapy instead of the initially planned VT ablation.

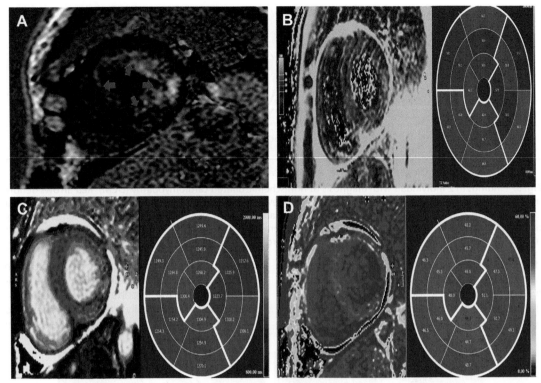

Fig. 7. CMR tissue characterization in a patient with nonischemic cardiomyopathy using 1.5 T scanner. (*A*) Global subendocardial LGE (*red arrows*) paired with abnormal contrast kinetics. (*B*) T2 mapping shows a diffusely elevated T2 value of 62 ms. (*C*) Native T1 mapping shows marked diffusely elevated T1 value of 1261 ms. (*D*) ECV map shows significant diffuse extracellular volume expansion (ECV value of 48%). Patient subsequently had an endomyocardial biopsy confirming diagnosis of AL amyloidosis.

its preclinical course, where steps might be taken to prevent SCD.

Phenotype-First Approach

Use of genotyping in suspected or phenotype indeterminate individuals can aid in establishing the correct diagnosis. It is important to recognize, however, that certain gene mutations still have undetermined significance, and gene-elusive forms of the hereditary ACM can have negative or inconclusive genetic testing, and a "negative genetic screening" should not exclude the possibility of ACM diagnosis.[10] Therefore, a personalized patient-specific approach that implements clinical assessment, detailed family history, diagnostic testing, and genetic counseling is needed to provide comprehensive patient care. CMR plays a central role in such an evaluation (**Fig. 10**).

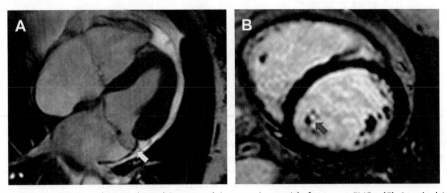

Fig. 8. CMR showing MVP and MAD (*A, white arrow*) in a patient with frequent PVCs. (*B*) Atypical LGE in the posteromedial papillary muscle (*red arrow*).

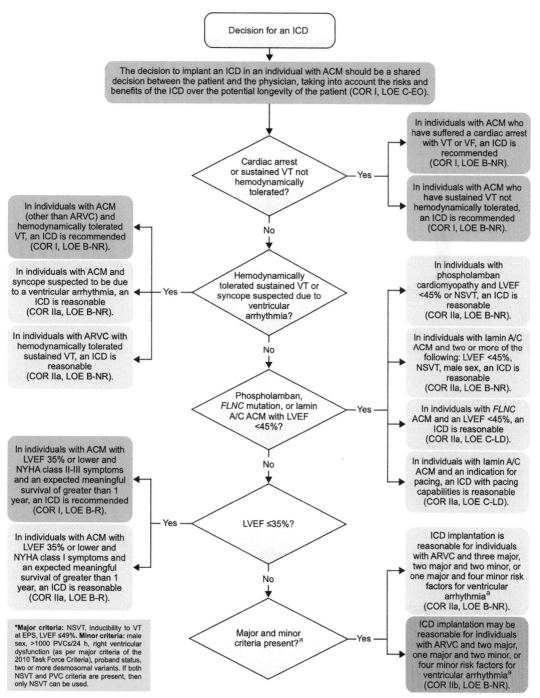

Fig. 9. Flowchart for implantable cardioverter defibrillator (ICD) decision-making in ACM per HRS expert consensus statement (2019). Green = class I recommendation, yellow = class IIa recommendation, orange = class IIb recommendation. COR, class of recommendation; EPS, electrophysiology studies; FLNC, filamin-C; LOE, level of evidence; LVEF, left ventricular ejection fraction; NSVT, nonsustained ventricular tachycardia; NYHA, New York Heart Association; PVC, premature ventricular contractions; VF, ventricular fibrillation; VT, ventricular tachycardia. (*From* Towbin JA, McKenna WJ, Abrams DJ, et al. 2019 HRS expert consensus statement on evaluation, risk stratification, and management of arrhythmogenic cardiomyopathy: Executive summary. Heart Rhythm. 2019;16(11):e373-e407.)

Phenotype-first approach

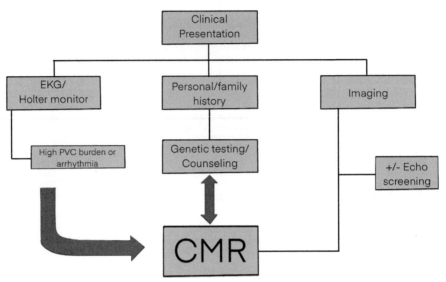

Fig. 10. Flowchart detailing phenotype-first approach for comprehensive assessment of ACM and the crucial role of CMR in such evaluation.

Genotype-first approach

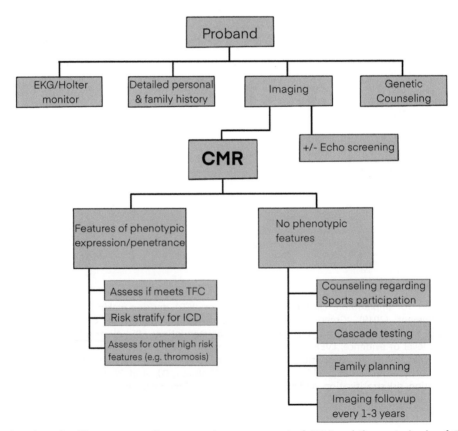

Fig. 11. Flowchart detailing genotype-first approach to assessment of ACM and the central role of CMR. ICD, implantable cardioverter defibrillator; TFC, task force criteria.

Genotype-First Approach

It has been reported that up to 16% of healthy individuals might carry missense gene mutations in one of the major ACM-related genes.[35] With expanding availability of genomic sequencing and personalized genetic testing, including direct-to-consumer testing, incidental identification of individuals with disease-causing genetic mutations is becoming more common. Moreover, over the past decade, population health initiative and research sequencing programs such as the UK BioBank,[36] Geisinger MyCode Community Health Initiative[37] (DiscovEHR cohort), and eMERGE9[38] have developed population-based genomic screening programs and are evaluating associated phenotypic expression of different genes.

The American College of Medical Genetics and Genomics also recommends reporting of incidental and secondary findings related to ACM from clinical genomic sequencing due to anticipated benefit.[39]

Multiple genetic variants associated with arrhythmogenic conditions are increasingly being considered clinically actionable and hence recommended for screening. Estimates of penetrance of these genetic mutations vary but have been reported to be as low as 6% according to one analysis.[40]

The clinical management of such "gene-first" probands remains challenging. Data from large

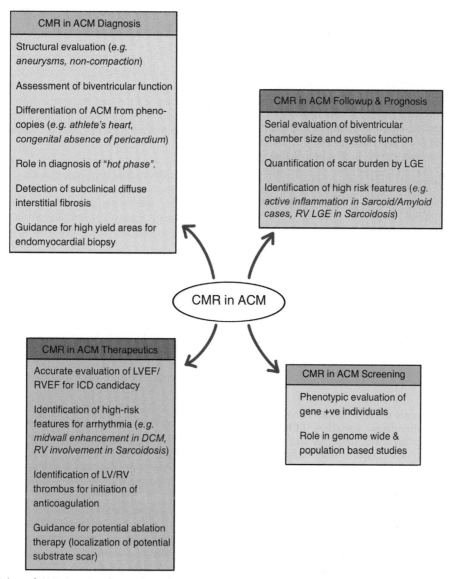

Fig. 12. Value of CMR in ACM diagnosis and management.

population-based Biobanks initiatives would hopefully provide further clues into the clinical significance of these genes and ideal clinical approach.

CMR can be a very useful tool in assessing phenotypic expression in probands and gene-positive family members by detecting low- or high-risk phenotypes and allowing for imaging-based prognostication to detect individuals who might benefit from preventative therapies (**Fig. 11**). Further research is needed to validate prognostic significance of these findings.

SUMMARY

ACM is a term that encompasses a wide variety of heterogeneous hereditary and nonhereditary disorders that can result in cardiac arrhythmias. Although the arrhythmic components of these conditions overlap, they vary greatly in clinical course and therapeutic approach.

Over the past few decades, significant strides have been made to better understand the underlying pathophysiology and disease process for these conditions enabling individualized patient-centric diagnosis and management approach.

The role of CMR is of paramount importance, as it plays an essential role in accurate initial diagnosis (**Fig. 12**) and assists in clinical decision-making and follow-up for affected individuals and families. Although the role of CMR has been highlighted in recent diagnostic criteria, it remains markedly underutilized.

Future research is needed to assess the value of advanced tissue characterization techniques in identifying patients with early subclinical phenotypes. There is also aspiration that MRI-driven data will be incorporated in future risk calculators for prediction of arrhythmias and guidance of therapy.

CLINICS CARE POINTS

- Underdiagnosis of ACM remains a challenge given its phenotypic variation. CMR use is essential for accurate diagnosis and to evaluate for high-risk features that might predispose to SCD.

- CMR is a useful tool for phenotypic evaluation of gene positive individuals who are identified as carriers of ACM-related gene mutations.

- Although management of asymptomatic subclinical gene carriers remains unclear, CMR is a useful tool for serial phenotypic evaluation.

DISCLOSURE

The authors have no conflict of interest to disclose in relation to the present work.

REFERENCES

1. Marcus FI, Fontaine GH, Guiraudon G, et al. Right ventricular dysplasia: a report of 24 adult cases. Circulation 1982;65(2):384–98.
2. Corrado D, Basso C. Arrhythmogenic left ventricular cardiomyopathy. Heart 2022;108(9):733–43.
3. McKenna WJ, Thiene G, Nava A, et al. Task Force of the Working Group Myocardial and Pericardial Disease of the European Society of Cardiology and of the Scientific Council on Cardiomyopathies of the International Society and Federation of Cardiology. Diagnosis of arrhythmogenic right ventricular dysplasia/cardiomyopathy. Br Heart J 1994;71(3):215–8.
4. Towbin JA, McKenna WJ, Abrams DJ, et al. HRS expert consensus statement on evaluation, risk stratification, and management of arrhythmogenic cardiomyopathy. Heart Rhythm 2019;16(11):e301–72.
5. Sabbag A, Essayagh B, Barrera JDR, et al. EHRA expert consensus statement on arrhythmic mitral valve prolapse and mitral annular disjunction complex in collaboration with the ESC Council on valvular heart disease and the European Association of Cardiovascular Imaging endorsed cby the Heart Rhythm Society, by the Asia Pacific Heart Rhythm Society, and by the Latin American Heart Rhythm Society. Europace 2022;24(12):1981–2003.
6. Te Riele AS, James CA, Philips B, et al. Mutation-positive arrhythmogenic right ventricular dysplasia/cardiomyopathy: the triangle of dysplasia displaced. J Cardiovasc Electrophysiol 2013;24(12):1311–20.
7. Cerrone M, Delmar M. Desmosomes and the sodium channel complex: implications for arrhythmogenic cardiomyopathy and Brugada syndrome. Trends Cardiovasc Med 2014;24(5):184–90.
8. Li GL, Saguner AM, Fontaine GH. Naxos disease: from the origin to today. Orphanet J Rare Dis 2018;13(1):1–11.
9. Patel V, Asatryan B, Siripanthong B, et al. State of the art review on genetics and precision medicine in arrhythmogenic cardiomyopathy. Int J Mol Sci 2020;21(18):6615.
10. Groeneweg JA, Bhonsale A, James CA, et al. Clinical presentation, long-term follow-up, and outcomes of 1001 arrhythmogenic right ventricular dysplasia/cardiomyopathy patients and family members. Circ Cardiovasc Genet 2015;8(3):437–46.
11. Marcus FI, Edson S, Towbin JA. Genetics of arrhythmogenic right ventricular cardiomyopathy: a practical guide for physicians. J Am Coll Cardiol 2013;61(19):1945–8.

12. Hulot JS, Jouven X, Empana JP, et al. Natural history and risk stratification of arrhythmogenic right ventricular dysplasia/cardiomyopathy. Circulation 2004; 110(14):1879–84.

13. Dalal D, Nasir K, Bomma C, et al. Arrhythmogenic right ventricular dysplasia: a United States experience. Circulation 2005;112(25):3823–32.

14. Haugaa KH, Haland TF, Leren IS, et al. Arrhythmogenic right ventricular cardiomyopathy, clinical manifestations, and diagnosis. EP Europace 2016;18(7): 965–72.

15. Carruth ED, Fielden S, Alsaid A, et al. Abstract 13159: Subclinical cardiac magnetic resonance imaging reveals subtle myocardial tissue abnormalities in individuals with arrhythmogenic cardiomyopathy-associated genetic variants. Circulation 2021; 144(Suppl_1). https://doi.org/10.1161/circ.144. suppl_1.13159.

16. Miles C, Finocchiaro G, Papadakis M, et al. Sudden death and left ventricular involvement in arrhythmogenic cardiomyopathy. Circulation 2019;139(15): 1786–97.

17. Meraviglia V, Alcalde M, Campuzano O, et al. Inflammation in the Pathogenesis of Arrhythmogenic Cardiomyopathy: Secondary Event or Active Driver? Front Cardiovasc Med 2021;8:784715. https://doi. org/10.3389/fcvm.2021.784715.

18. Asatryan B, Asimaki A, Landstrom AP, et al. Inflammation and Immune Response in Arrhythmogenic Cardiomyopathy: State-of-the-Art Review. Circulation 2021;144(20):1646–55.

19. Bariani R, Rigato I, Cipriani A, et al. Myocarditis-like Episodes in Patients with Arrhythmogenic Cardiomyopathy: A Systematic Review on the So-Called Hot-Phase of the Disease. Biomolecules 2022;12(9). https://doi.org/10.3390/biom12091324.

20. Marcus FI, McKenna WJ, Sherrill D, et al. Diagnosis of arrhythmogenic right ventricular cardiomyopathy/ dysplasia: proposed modification of the task force criteria. Circulation 2010;121(13):1533–41.

21. Corrado D, Marra MP, Zorzi A, et al. Diagnosis of arrhythmogenic cardiomyopathy: the Padua criteria. Int J Cardiol 2020;319:106–14.

22. Malik N, Mukherjee M, Wu KC, et al. Multimodality Imaging in Arrhythmogenic Right Ventricular Cardiomyopathy. Circ Cardiovasc Imaging 2022;15(2): e013725.

23. Dawson DK, Hawlisch K, Prescott G, et al. Prognostic role of CMR in patients presenting with ventricular arrhythmias. JACC Cardiovasc Imaging 2013;6(3):335–44.

24. Czimbalmos C, Csecs I, Dohy Z, et al. Cardiac magnetic resonance based deformation imaging: role of feature tracking in athletes with suspected arrhythmogenic right ventricular cardiomyopathy. Int J Cardiovasc Imaging 2019;35(3): 529–38.

25. Halliday BP, Gulati A, Ali A, et al. Association between midwall late gadolinium enhancement and sudden cardiac death in patients with dilated cardiomyopathy and mild and moderate left ventricular systolic dysfunction. Circulation 2017;135(22): 2106–15.

26. Athwal PSS, Chhikara S, Ismail MF, et al. Cardiovascular Magnetic Resonance Imaging Phenotypes and Long-term Outcomes in Patients With Suspected Cardiac Sarcoidosis. JAMA cardiology 2022;7(10):1057–66.

27. Amano Y, Tachi M, Tani H, et al. T2-weighted cardiac magnetic resonance imaging of edema in myocardial diseases. Sci World J 2012;2012.

28. Maceira AM, Joshi J, Prasad SK, et al. Cardiovascular magnetic resonance in cardiac amyloidosis. Circulation 2005;111(2):186–93.

29. Perea RJ, Ortiz-Perez JT, Sole M, et al. T1 mapping: characterisation of myocardial interstitial space. Insights Imaging 2015;6(2):189–202.

30. Martinez-Naharro A, Abdel-Gadir A, Treibel TA, et al. CMR-Verified Regression of Cardiac AL Amyloid After Chemotherapy. JACC Cardiovasc Imaging 2018; 11(1):152–4.

31. Corrado D, Wichter T, Link MS, et al. Treatment of arrhythmogenic right ventricular cardiomyopathy/ dysplasia: an international task force consensus statement. Circulation 2015;132(5):441–53.

32. Cadrin-Tourigny J, Bosman LP, Nozza A, et al. A new prediction model for ventricular arrhythmias in arrhythmogenic right ventricular cardiomyopathy. Eur Heart J 2022;43(32):e1–9.

33. Dickfeld T, Kato R, Zviman M, et al. Characterization of radiofrequency ablation lesions with gadolinium-enhanced cardiovascular magnetic resonance imaging. J Am Coll Cardiol 2006;47(2):370–8.

34. Dickfeld T, Tian J, Ahmad G, et al. MRI-Guided ventricular tachycardia ablation: integration of late gadolinium-enhanced 3D scar in patients with implantable cardioverter-defibrillators. Circ Arrhythm Electrophysiol 2011;4(2):172–84.

35. Kapplinger JD, Landstrom AP, Salisbury BA, et al. Distinguishing arrhythmogenic right ventricular cardiomyopathy/dysplasia-associated mutations from background genetic noise. J Am Coll Cardiol 2011;57(23):2317–27.

36. Hylind RJ, Pereira AC, Quiat D, et al. Population prevalence of premature truncating variants in plakophilin-2 and association with arrhythmogenic right ventricular cardiomyopathy: A UK Biobank analysis. Circ Genom Precis Med 2022;15(3): e003507.

37. Carey DJ, Fetterolf SN, Davis FD, et al. The Geisinger MyCode community health initiative: an electronic health record–linked biobank for precision medicine research. Genet Med 2016;18(9): 906–13.

38. Jarvik GP, Amendola LM, Berg JS, et al. Return of genomic results to research participants: the floor, the ceiling, and the choices in between. Am J Hum Genet 2014;94(6):818–26.

39. Kalia SS, Adelman K, Bale SJ, et al. Recommendations for reporting of secondary findings in clinical exome and genome sequencing, 2016 update (ACMG SF v2.0): a policy statement of the American College of Medical Genetics and Genomics. Genet Med 2017;19(2):249–55.

40. Carruth ED, Young W, Beer D, et al. Prevalence and Electronic Health Record-Based Phenotype of Loss-of-Function Genetic Variants in Arrhythmogenic Right Ventricular Cardiomyopathy-Associated Genes. Circ Genom Precis Med 2019;12(11): e002579.

Viral Myocarditis and Dilated Cardiomyopathy as a Consequence—Changing Insights from Advanced Imaging

Nicolas Kang, MD[a], Matthias G. Friedrich, MD[b,c], Dmitry Abramov, MD[d],
Ana Martinez-Naharro, MD[e], Marianna Fontana, MD, PhD[e],
Purvi Parwani, MBBS, MPH[d,*]

KEYWORDS

- Viral myocarditis • Nonischemic cardiomyopathy • Dilated cardiomyopathy
- Cardiac magnetic resonance

KEY POINTS

- Viral myocarditis involves viral-induced myocyte necrosis and inflammation, detectable through immunohistopathology and CMR, which highlight tissue damage and inflammation, aiding in diagnosis and risk stratification.
- Advanced CMR imaging can detect myocardial inflammation and tissue changes characteristic of myocarditis, aiding in diagnosis, prognosis, and determining treatment approaches.
- The revised Lake Louise Criteria use CMR measurements of T1, T2, and extracellular volume, improving diagnostic accuracy. Late gadolinium enhancement is a outcome predictor.
- CMR findings in COVID-19 patients sparked debates on whether these represent true myocarditis or other forms of cardiac injury due to systemic inflammation.
- Future myocarditis imaging advances aim for enhanced specificity in diagnosing viral myocarditis, better risk stratification, and more effective monitoring of disease progression and recovery.

[a] Department of Medicine, Loma Linda University Medical Center, 11234 Anderson Street, Loma Linda, CA 92354, USA; [b] Department of Medicine, McGill University Health Centre, 1001 Decarie Boulevard, Montreal, Quebec H4A 3J1, Canada; [c] Department of Diagnostic Radiology, McGill University Health Centre, Montreal, Quebec, Canada; [d] Division of Cardiology, Loma Linda University Medical Center, 11234 Anderson Street, Loma Linda, CA 92354, USA; [e] UCL CMR Department at the Royal Free Hospital and the National Amyloidosis Centre, University College, London
* Corresponding author. Loma Linda University Medical Center, Loma Linda, CA 92354.
E-mail address: pparwani@llu.edu
Twitter: @purviparwani (P.P.)

Heart Failure Clin 19 (2023) 445–459
https://doi.org/10.1016/j.hfc.2023.03.009

OBJECTIVES

- Describe the pathophysiology of viral myocarditis and its correlation to abnormalities seen on immunohistopathology and quantitative cardiac magnetic resonance (CMR).

- Explain how advanced imaging can guide the diagnosis and management of viral myocarditis.

- Understand the updated Lake Louise Criteria and the parametric markers that predict outcomes in myocarditis.

- Describe the controversies surrounding coronavirus disease 2019-related abnormalities in CMR.

- Understand the applications of future developments in myocarditis imaging.

INTRODUCTION

Viral myocarditis is a nonischemic myocardial inflammation after viral infection, leading to myocardial injury, possible cardiac dysfunction, and life-threatening arrhythmias. Presentations are highly variable in severity and course, with a broad differential, making diagnosis difficult. Viral myocarditis is a common cause of acute myocarditis (AM), primarily a mild and self-limited disease presenting with chest pain and dyspnea for less than 1 month, troponin elevations, and electrocardiographic abnormalities. Nearly 25% of cases may develop prolonged inflammation and persistent myocardial dysfunction, as in inflammatory cardiomyopathy (ICMP). However, up to 25% can progress to acute decompensation or dilated cardiomyopathy (DCM), which predicts a 40% mortality rate at 10 years.[1] Initial evaluation with cardiac troponins, inflammatory markers, electrocardiogram, and echocardiography can raise suspicion for AM but none is diagnostic for AM as a standalone test. Coronary angiography or other ischemic evaluation is generally pursued to exclude acute coronary syndrome (ACS) when the pretest probability of ACS is high.[2] Although endomyocardial biopsy (EMB) remains the gold standard for the diagnosis of hemodynamically unstable AM, cardiac magnetic resonance (CMR) is the diagnostic test of choice for stable AM and offers excellent diagnostic accuracy, tissue characterization, risk stratification, and identification of high-risk features for poor cardiac outcomes, including DCM and sudden cardiac death (SCD).[1] This review will discuss the pathophysiology of viral myocarditis, how it guides diagnostic evaluation, and how multiparametric CMR improves the risk stratification and management of viral myocarditis.

PATHOPHYSIOLOGY

The acute inflammatory phase of viral myocarditis often lasts 1 to 3 days and is associated with viral replication-induced myocyte necrosis. Myocardial injury can be induced by cardiotropic (adenoviruses, enteroviruses), vasculotropic (parvovirus B19 [PVB19]), lymphotropic (cytomegalovirus, Epstein–Barr virus, human herpesvirus 6 [HHV6]), cardiotoxic (hepatitis C virus, HIV, influenza), and angiotensin II (ACE2)-tropic viruses (coronaviridae). Injured myocytes release intracellular antigens, which stimulate proinflammatory cytokine release, vascular hyperemia, myocardial edema, infiltration of monocytes, and activation of the adaptive immune response. Although most cases of acute myocardial inflammation resolve spontaneously within 1 month, myocyte injury may perpetuate the immunologic response for months despite undetectable levels of viral genome as seen in chronic postviral autoimmune myocarditis. Additionally, severe inflammation can produce extensive myocyte injury, necrosis, fibrosis, and gap junction disruption, presenting clinically as myocardial dysfunction, structural abnormalities, and arrhythmias.[3,4]

PATHOLOGIC GUIDANCE FOR MYOCARDITIS

Using the Dallas Criteria, EMB with inflammatory infiltrates and nonischemic myocyte necrosis remains the reference gold standard for definitively diagnosing unstable myocarditis.[5–7] However, EMB is invasive and complicates 1% to 9% of cases, depending on the procedure volume. EMB also has high sampling error, lower sensitivity with conventional hematoxylin-eosin staining, and lower specificity compared with CMR, as seen in **Table 1**.[8,9] Although sensitivity can increase with multiple samples, biventricular testing, and immunohistochemistry, EMB is reserved for severe forms of myocarditis as follows: AM with severe heart failure or myocardial dysfunction, shock, ventricular arrhythmias (VA), and high-grade atrioventricular blocks; AM or ICMP with eosinophilia, chronic, or relapsing myocardial injury.[2,8]

EMB-confirmed myocarditis requires immunohistochemistry and viral polymerase chain reaction to define the inflammatory cells and responsible pathogen.[10] Although ESC recommends characterizing the inflammation and viral persistence to guide treatment options, there are no robust clinical trials to guide pathogen-directed therapy effectively.[2]

IMAGING GUIDANCE FOR MYOCARDITIS

Echocardiography is the best initial imaging test for evaluating suspected AM and can identify other

Table 1
Diagnostic tests for evaluating acute myocarditis with radiographic features, sensitivity, specificity, prognostics, and limitations

Diagnostic Test	Diagnostic Features of AM	Sensitivity	Specificity	Prognostic Markers	Limitations
Biventricular EMB[36,37]	Myocardial infiltration with leukocytes. PCR detects viral genome in myocytes	54.2%	64.3%	+ Dallas criteria: independently predicts death and orthotopic heart transplantation (OHT) Inflammatory infiltrates: HR 3.5 for cardiac death and OHT	Invasive, low sensitivity, sampling error, high false-negative rate
Tnp T[38-40]	Myocardial injury: Elevation above 99th percentile URL	100%	69%	None	Absent tissue characterization, cannot differentiate ischemic from nonischemic myocardial injury
ECG[41,42]	ST-elevation, T-wave inversion, PQ-depression, and QT-prolongation	47%	77%	Atrial fibrillation, BBB, ischemic changes, QT-prolongation, and heart rate >120 are associated with increased mortality	Low sensitivity, low specificity, absent tissue characterization
CKMB[40]	Elevated serum CKMB above URL	6%	100%	None	Low sensitivity, absent tissue characterization
Echo[2,43]	Low LVEF, wall motion abnormalities, increased LV thickness, and LV dilatation	-	-	Low LVEF: independent predictor of mortality Biventricular dysfunction at initial presentation: independent predictor of mortality and OHT	Poor tissue characterization, not sufficient for diagnosis as a standalone test
Updated LLC[11]	Edema on T2, nonischemic myocardial injury on T1, pericarditis, systolic LV dysfunction	80%	88%	See later discussion	CMR is effective for diagnosing AM only when clinical suspicion is high, is unable to determine underlying cause of myocarditis, has slow throughput, and may not be feasible in hemodynamically unstable cases

(continued on next page)

Table 1
(continued)

Diagnostic Test	Diagnostic Features of AM	Sensitivity	Specificity	Prognostic Markers	Limitations
T2 mapping[15]	Global or regional increase in T2 relaxation time	78%	84%	T2 intensity: predicts worse outcomes, heart failure, and higher MACE[33]; Persistent T2 intensity: predicts persistent LV dysfunction[33]	Similar to T1. Less sensitive for detecting edema in myocarditis with chronic symptoms than T2
ECV[15]	Increased myocardial ECV derived from T1-mapping	75%	76%	Increased ECV: associated with higher MACE[44]	Inferior diagnostic accuracy compared with native T1-mapping. Sensitivity for edema decreases after 2 wk of symptoms
LGE[15]	Increased LGE signal typically in subepicardial or midmyocardial regions	69%	96%	LGE presence: all-cause mortality (HR 3–8),[28,29] cardiac mortality (HR 13),[28] SCD (HR 14)[26]; Midwall, anteroseptal, patchy distribution: associated with increased mortality[22,45]; Increased LGE extent: worse outcomes, lower LVEF, RV function, higher MACE[31,46]; Persistent LGE at 6 mo: higher RR than no LGE[31]; Midmyocardial LGE and LGE without edema: worse prognosis; LGE without edema is associated with VA and SCD[31,33]	Absence of baseline CMR and LGE can make new or chronic LGE difficult to distinguish

Abbreviations: AM, acute myocarditis; BBB, bundle branch block; CKMB, creatine kinase-myocardial band; CMR, cardiac magnetic resonance; cTn, cardiac troponin; ECG, electrocardiogram; ECV, extracellular volume; HR, hazard ratio; LGE, late gadolinium enhancement; LLC, Lake Louise Criteria; LV, left ventricular; MACE, major acute cardiovascular events; OHT, orthotopic heart transplantation; PCR, polymerase chain reaction; RV, right ventricular; SCD, sudden cardiac death; TnP, troponin; URL, upper reference limit; VA, ventricular arrhythmias.

causes of heart failure (valvular disease, congenital heart disease, or cardiomyopathy), wall motion abnormalities, and pericardial effusion.[3] However, echocardiographic findings of acute and chronic myocarditis alone are nonspecific and cannot accurately diagnose myocarditis.[2]

However, CMR can play an important role in diagnosing AM due to its excellent sensitivity for detecting and monitoring pathologic tissue changes, including hyperemia, edema, extracellular debris, myocyte injury, necrosis, and fibrosis. Although CMR abnormalities cannot identify the specific cause of AM, advancements during the last decade significantly improved the diagnostic performance, tissue characterization, and prognostication using CMR for stable AM within 4 weeks of symptom onset.[1,11–17] Guidelines endorse CMR before EMB to diagnose and monitor stable AM[2,10]; identify suspected myocarditis in heart failure,[18] valvular, and pericardial disease[19]; differentiate ischemic from nonischemic myocardial injury[19]; exclude nonischemic injury in ischemia with nonobstructive coronary arteries[20]; and determine the presence and extent of myopericardial inflammation and fibrosis.[22] Additionally, CMR can exclude conditions whose presentations may overlap with myocarditis, including infiltrative cardiomyopathies, which may significantly alter the course of care.

Several studies propose LGE patterns may suggest the underlying viral type. In one small study of 81 EMB-confirmed viral myocarditis with LGE, Marholdt and colleagues reported radiographically distinct phenotypes that depended on the type of virus.[21] For example, among PVB19 myocarditis cases (n = 49), 94% had LGE, all with a subepicardial distribution that involved the inferior and lateral walls and healed on follow-up CMR. Among HHV6 myocarditis (n = 16), all had LGE with a midmyocardial distribution in the anteroseptal location that was persistent but significantly decreased on follow-up CMR. Among the 80% of HHV6/PVB19 myocarditis (n = 15) with LGE, 95% had a midmyocardial, striae distribution that persisted without significant improvement or worsened on follow-up CMR. In the study, HHV6/PVB19 myocarditis was an independent predictor of persistent ventricular dysfunction and was also more likely to have malaise, fatigue, bundle branch block, and insidious onset heart failure (ie, dyspnea and peripheral edema) for a median of 21 days before initial presentation. Aquaro and colleagues reported a similar distribution of LGE patterns and noted a midmyocardial involvement in the anteroseptal location had worse outcomes than other CMR patterns.[22] In another small study of suspected influenza A-related myocarditis with

myocardial inflammation on CMR (n = 2), all had global myocardial edema on T2-weighted imaging with midmyocardial LGE located in the septum and inferior left ventricular (LV).[23]

DIAGNOSTIC MARKERS OF ACUTE MYOCARDITIS USING MULTIPARAMETRIC CARDIAC MAGNETIC RESONANCE

The original 2009 Lake Louise Criteria (LLC) combined 3 CMR techniques to diagnose suspected AM if 2 out of the 3 following findings were present: myocardial edema (T2-weighted imaging), hyperemia (early gadolinium enhancement [EGE] on T1-weighted images), and fibrosis or scar (late gadolinium enhancement [LGE]).[24] Lagan and colleagues reported in a 2017 meta-analysis a diagnostic accuracy of 83% (sensitivity 80%, specificity 87%). However, limitations existed. First, T2-weighted spin-echo images have low signal-to-noise ratios and were not sufficiently sensitive to detect regional edema with milder inflammation when present on 36% of EMB-positive AM. Second, the qualitative analysis relied on visualizing relative signal intensities in the region of interest, making homogenous myocardial inflammation detection more difficult.[11] Third, detecting edema and EGE required fast spin-echo sequences, prone to motion artifacts with irregular breathing and heart rates.[24] Although suffering from similar shortcomings, quantitative T1, T2, and extracellular volume (ECV) measurements, for the most part, alleviate these limitations by decreasing reliance on qualitative detection of relative signal changes, offering short-breath-hold acquisition sequences, and detecting homogenous tissue edema with greater sensitivity and reliability. **Table 1** shows the diagnostic performance of each CMR parameter discussed in the following section as reported in a meta-analysis by Kotanidis and colleagues.[15]

Quantitative T1 and T2 mapping detects myocardial edema and displays pixel-wise measurements of the prolonged myocardial relaxation times caused by an increased tissue water content.[18,25] T1-values and T1-derived ECV increase with edema, hyperemia, and more chronic changes (ie, fibrosis and necrosis), as seen in DCM. The MyoRacer Trial reported that native T1-mapping yielded the highest diagnostic accuracy (81%; sensitivity 88%, specificity 67%) among all parameters in myocarditis patients with symptoms less than 14 days but sensitivity and diagnostic accuracy declined sharply (45%, sensitivity 27%, specificity 94%) in patients with symptoms greater than 14 days. The diagnostic accuracy of ECV was also higher for patients with acute symptoms (75%, sensitivity 75%, specificity 72%) than for chronic symptoms (67%, sensitivity 69%, specificity 61%). Thus, when inflammation is prolonged, both T1 and ECV lose their ability to discriminate between edema in AM and more chronic tissue changes and may reflect a diseased myocardium.[11,13] Conversely, T2-mapping may be more sensitive to detecting edema, irrespective of fibrosis. In the same study, T2-mapping was the only parameter with acceptable diagnostic accuracy in patients with acute (80%, sensitivity 85%, specificity 68%) and chronic (73%, sensitivity 71%, specificity 88%) symptoms.[13] Hence, only T2-mapping can differentiate edema in chronic myocarditis from noninflammatory DCM.

More LGE accumulates inside injured myocytes and the extracellular space when severe inflammation causes necrosis and scarring. As inflammation wanes and scars contract, LGE intensifies while markers for acute inflammation (ie, T2 intensity) resolve.[11] A pooled meta-analysis of patients with infarct-like AM showed LGE was the most useful diagnostic finding (diagnostic accuracy 92%, sensitivity 86%, and specificity 100%). Still, sensitivity decreased with mild inflammation and subtle necrosis.[11] Although LGE is not specific for acute inflammation and cannot distinguish active from resolved myocarditis, it can identify the mechanism of myocardial injury, grade inflammation severity when more severe, and predict clinical outcomes. For example, myocarditis characteristically demonstrates a patchy, subepicardial, and midmyocardial LGE pattern that favors the basal and midinferolateral walls and extends to the subendocardium with severe inflammation; in contrast, ischemic injury shows subendocardial or transmural LGE.[11]

Supportive criteria include myocardial dysfunction and pericarditis but neither alone is sensitive nor specific enough to diagnose AM. On CMR, myocardial dysfunction shows global or regional hypokinesis, wall motion abnormalities, or reduced ejection fraction but these are not always present in AM and may result from other causes.[11] Myocardial and pericardial inflammation frequently coexist; however, cine images are not specific enough to distinguish myocarditis from noninflammatory myocardial disease. More specific findings of pericardial inflammation include pericardial thickening on T1-weighted images, abnormal LGE, and hyperintensity on native T2, T1, and T2 mapping.

UPDATED LAKE LOUISE CRITERIA

The updated LLC adds T1 and T2 mapping to the sequences to identify nonischemic myocardial

injury and myocardial edema, respectively, and diagnose AM in highly suspected cases with excellent diagnostic accuracy.[11] Major criteria are based on edema by T2 (eg, global or regional increase in T2 relaxation time or T2-weighted signal intensity) and nonischemic myocardial injury by T1 (eg, T1 hyperintensity, increased ECV, or LGE), whereas supportive criteria are visualized on cine sequences and include pericarditis (eg, effusion, abnormal LGE, T2, or T1) and systolic LV dysfunction (eg, regional or global wall motion abnormalities), as seen in **Fig. 1**. Although AM is diagnosed with higher specificity with 2 major criteria, the updated LLC supports a diagnosis of AM with one major criterion (positive T1-based or T2-based marker) with a supportive clinical presentation or one supportive criterion.[11]

After adopting the original LLC, studies explored various combinations of CMR-based myocarditis markers to improve diagnostic accuracy further while maximizing sensitivity over specificity. Chu and colleagues[11] showed that removing EGE from the original LLC did not worsen the diagnostic performance. Mapping sequences also added theoretic benefits to native T1 and T2, as discussed previously. Several 2-out-of-2 combinations outperformed the median diagnostic accuracy of classic LLC (84%), namely T2-weighted imaging with LGE (90%), T2-mapping with LGE (86%), and the contrast-free T2-mapping with T1-mapping (84%). T2 mapping with ECV may also theoretically be beneficial for evaluating AM with global edema but large prospective trials are lacking. Although T1-mapping with LGE also outperformed the original LLC, studies do not yet support T1 can distinguish acute and chronic myocarditis.[11]

PROGNOSTIC MARKERS FOR MYOCARDITIS USING MULTIPARAMETRIC CARDIAC MAGNETIC RESONANCE

Aside from its essential diagnostic role, CMR can characterize tissues, which allows superior risk stratification compared with other well-known markers of poor outcomes, including reduced left ventricular ejection fraction (LVEF) and higher New York Heart Association (NYHA) functional class.[26–28] Current evidence suggests that LGE presence, location (anteroseptal, midmyocardial), distribution (patchy), and extent were all strong markers for adverse outcomes in viral AM and may represent a nidus for malignant arrhythmias. Currently, LGE presence is the strongest independent predictor of adverse outcomes in viral AM, including all-cause mortality, cardiac death, and SCD but biventricular dysfunction at initial

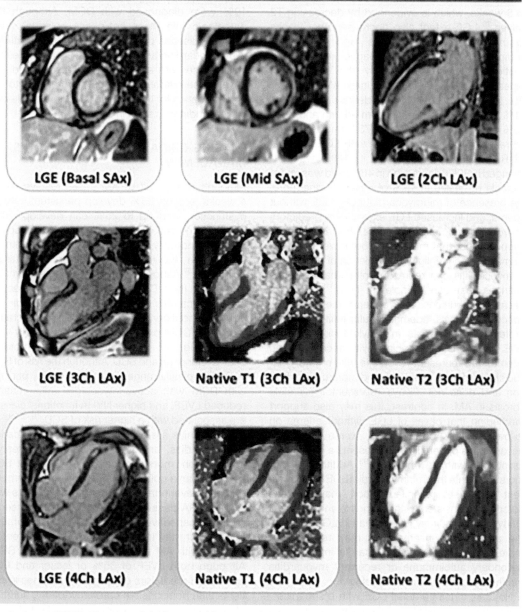

Fig. 1. Acute COVID-19 myocarditis diagnosed by CMR. This figure shows an example of CMR, showing extensive subendocardial and midmyocardial LGE and elevated T1 and T2 mapping values involving all LV segments. The top panel illustrates the LGE involving all LV segments in the short-axis and long-axis views. The middle and bottom panels show LGE, elevated T1, and T2 signal values extensively involving the LV myocardium. 2Ch, 2 chamber; 3Ch, 3 chamber; 4Ch, 4 chamber; LAx, long axis; LGE, late-gadolinium enhancement; SAx, short axis.

presentation was a leading predictor of mortality and heart transplantation.[2,26,28,29] **Table 1** summarizes the diagnostic and prognostic markers for AM discussed previously.

Follow-up with repeat CMR is important for assessing functional recovery and prognosis in AM. Edema and inflammation usually resolve in 4 to 6 weeks, which is evidenced by decreasing T2 values.[30] LGE extent also decreases over weeks to months in most cases and may heal completely.[31] Aquaro and colleagues reported in a multicenter prospective study the benefits of repeating CMR 6 months after initial AM presentation. In this study, most (84%) edema was resolved, 11% had complete healing from edema and LGE, 16% had LGE and edema, and 73% had LGE alone on repeat CMR. Among those with LGE on initial CMR, LGE extent increased in 10%, was unchanged in 30%, decreased in 46%, and was undetectable or healed in 10% of cases. Furthermore, the presence of midmyocardial LGE, LGE without edema, and increased LGE extent were predictors of worse outcomes. Although LGE in MI strongly supports scar that may shrink but never resolves, a small but nonnegligible prevalence of acute LGE in myocarditis can represent inflammatory tissue changes that can completely heal.[31,32] This is because conditions that expand the interstitial space (ie, fibrosis, edema, cellular infiltration, and protein deposition, as in amyloidosis) produce LGE. Hence, LGE, especially with accompanying edema, can represent reversible inflammatory tissue changes such as edema and monocyte infiltration and does not always represent irreversible fibrosis in AM. In contrast, this may also support the finding that cases of LGE without edema on follow-up CMR portended a worse prognosis because this pattern likely represents a scar that is associated with VA and SCD.[33] Additionally, authors speculate that midmyocardial LGE may represent more severe inflammation that worsens outcomes, consistent with findings in another small study.[21,31] Intriguingly, the increased LGE extent in the absence of inflammation may represent a more subtle and ongoing myocardial injury from a secondary autoimmune or recurrent myocarditis but the exact mechanism is unclear.[31]

Notably, circumferential LGE with a subepicardial or midmyocardial ring-like pattern is a strong independent predictor of malignant arrhythmias in patients with nonsustained ventricular tachycardia (VT) and DCM with hazard ratio (HR) of 69 and 10, respectively, for combined outcomes (all-cause death, resuscitated arrest, VA, and implantable cardioverter-defibrillator [ICD] implantation).[34,35] Although described in case reports of myocarditis, the prognostic implication of ringed LGE in AM is not well studied. Arrhythmogenic cardiomyopathy (ACM) also increases the risk for VA and SCD. In 2022, Bariani and colleagues systematically reviewed 103 ACM patients who had a hot-phase episode (ie, chest pain, troponin elevation, electrocardiographic changes).[34] On hot-phase presentation, 26% were diagnosed with myocarditis, and 19% were diagnosed with DCM. Although the pathologic role these hot-phase episodes have on ACM disease progression is unclear, patients with myocarditis and a ringed LGE pattern, especially those with sustained or nonsustained VT, have worse outcome and need further monitoring and evaluation for ICD. A case of ACM with relevant clinical findings is seen in **Fig. 2**.

IMAGING GUIDANCE FOR MYOCARDITIS MANAGEMENT

Although nearly half of AM cases resolve within 4 weeks, around 25% develop persistent cardiac dysfunction, and up to 25% can develop either acute deterioration, DCM requiring heart transplantation, or mortality.[2] Symptomatic patients with LV dysfunction should be treated per heart failure guidelines.[47] Although non-steroidal anti-inflammatory drugs (NSAIDs) are fundamental for treating acute pericarditis, guidelines suggest avoiding it for AM without pericarditis because it may increase mortality.[2] DCM presentations are also highly variable ranging from no symptoms to overt symptoms of LV dysfunction and SCD. Although the risk of SCD in DCM typically ranges from 2% to 3%, patients with DCM with active myocardial inflammation, reduced LVEF, and higher NYHA functional classes are associated with a higher risk of SCD.[18,48,49]

Arrhythmias are another common complication of myocarditis, and it is managed with lifestyle modification, monitoring, and prevention of SCD per arrhythmia guidelines. Guidelines recommend primary prevention ICD placement in patients with DCM, NYHA class II-IV, and LVEF 35% or lesser. A recent prospective study showed incorporating LGE extent may improve the risk assessment of patients with AM for primary prevention of SCD. Although both LVEF of 35% or lesser and LGE are known predictors of adverse outcomes in patients with nonischemic cardiomyopathy, addition of LGE extent to primary prevention ICD evaluation improved prognostication, all-cause mortality, cardiac mortality, and SCD. Conversely, the addition of LVEF of 35% or lesser had no association to SCD.[63] As previously mentioned, myocarditis with ringed LGE should be strongly considered for primary ICD evaluation.

Repeat CMR offers prognostic implications that may alter management of myocarditis. Although

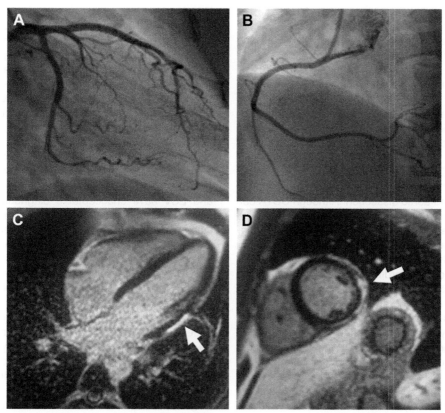

Fig. 2. AM in a case of ACM. A 20-year-old man with a family history of ICD placement in mother and SCD in cousin at the age of 28 years presented with chest pain, significantly elevated troponin T of 2.6 ng/mL, and sinus bradycardia on electrocardiogram. Coronary angiography revealed (*A, B*) nonobstructive coronaries, and CMR suggested AM given the subepicardial LGE (*C, white arrow*) along the inferolateral wall (*D, white arrow*).

CMR is typically repeated 3 to 6 months after initial evaluation, no consensus recommendation informs the exact timing. Athletes recently diagnosed with AM should avoid competitive and leisure sports while active inflammation is present. Because the duration of inflammation can vary, guidelines recommend avoiding moderate-to-high intensity exercise for 3 to 6 months, depending on the presence of edema on T2-weighted images and LGE on CMR.[51–53] In addition to repeat evaluation with troponins, inflammatory biomarkers, echocardiography, Holter monitoring, and exercise stress testing, CMR should be repeated, especially if edema or LGE was present during the acute illness.[17,54] Athletes should consider return to sports if they have normal troponins, inflammatory markers, LVEF, good functional capacity, and no evidence of acute inflammation on CMR or malignant arrhythmias during exercise testing.[51,55,56]

Imaging correlates with coronavirus disease 2019 (COVID-19)-associated and other viral myocarditis.

All clinically suspected cases of myocarditis should receive echocardiography at presentation and have repeated assessments when hemodynamics worsen.[2] This can help exclude noninflammatory cardiomyopathy assess cardiac function (eg, detect significant regional or global systolic LV dysfunction) and structure (eg, chamber size, wall thickness, wall motion abnormalities, pericardial effusion), and provide prognostication.[2] However, echocardiographic abnormalities are neither specific nor sensitive for diagnosing AM because they may be seen in other noninflammatory cardiomyopathies or be frequently absent in AM, respectively.[2] Dweck and colleagues reported in a large, perspective, multicenter study that 55% of suspected COVID-19 infections had echocardiographic abnormalities similar to other severe respiratory viral infections (ie, adenoviruses, enteroviruses, influenza A, B, and other coronaviridae),[57] namely LV dysfunction (39%), RV dysfunction (33%), and rarely myocarditis (3%), myocardial infarction (MI; 3%), and Takotsubo syndrome (TS; 2%).[58] Importantly, echocardiography directly changed the management in 33% of cases, including the level of care, disease-specific therapy (ie, heart failure, pulmonary embolism [PE], MI), and titration of hemodynamic support.[58]

Due to the propensity for arterial and venous thromboembolism, COVID-19 infections may present with myocardial injury, requiring multimodal imaging assessment to exclude ACS-like syndromes (ie, MI, PE, aortic dissection, TS, and myocarditis).[59] Especially in cases with myocardial injury and elevated D-dimer, coronary CT angiography (CCTA) has excellent negative predictive value (95%–100%) for excluding atherothrombotic MI, PE, and aortic dissection. Although CCTA can detect necrosis and fibrosis with delayed iodine contrast enhancement, it cannot effectively identify myocardial edema of myocarditis.[60] Thus, patients with high clinical suspicion for COVID-19-associated myocarditis should instead receive diagnostic evaluation with CMR by the updated LLC after excluding atherothrombotic MI.

Studies have also suggested that COVID-19-related myocarditis more often had LGE located in the inferior or inferoseptal wall with a right ventricular predilection. This pattern may be confounded by baseline cardiac comorbidities and can be atypical findings in 30% of healthy, asymptomatic athletes.[61] Ultimately, these factors may overestimate the prevalence of this pattern in studies without properly matched controls. It is worth restating that although CMR can offer excellent tissue characterization in patients with highly suspected AM, it is unable to determine the underlying viral cause without EMB, immunohistochemistry, and viral PCR with the available research.[11,13]

Furthermore, CMR abnormalities should be interpreted in the setting of myocarditis with high clinical suspicion for active inflammation. Several studies drew concern about COVID-19-related myocardial injury. Ng and colleagues reported abnormalities on CMR obtained 2 weeks or more (median 56 days of convalescence) after discharge in 16 patients who were asymptomatic (69%) or had cough, dyspnea, or mild chest pain (31%). In this retrospective cohort, CMR was abnormal in 56%, whereas 19% had nonischemic LGE and elevated T2. In a prospective study of 100 patients, Puntmann and colleagues reported abnormalities in 78% of CMR obtained 71 days after initial COVID positivity, and the majority had mild-to-moderate symptoms (49%) and without troponin elevations (85%). Pericardial enhancement was common (22%). Additionally, although there was more hyperintense T1-mapping in post-COVID-19 cases, T2-mapping, a more sensitive marker for edema when symptoms last greater than 14 days, was similar to controls, and nonischemic injury

(32%) was more common than nonischemic injury (20%). CMR abnormalities were also more prevalent in those with elevated troponin. This finding was supported by another study by Joy and colleagues who reported 74 health-care workers with mild to no symptoms for COVID-19 had a similar prevalence of abnormalities as healthy controls on CMR obtained 6 months postinfection. Although these results may seem that convalescent COVID-19 is often associated with CMR abnormalities found in myocarditis, the diagnostic accuracy of LLC in patients with low pretest probability for AM is not well known. Furthermore, both T1 and ECV have unacceptable diagnostic performance and poor sensitivity for detecting active inflammation when symptoms last greater than 14 days.[11,13] Hence, CMR abnormalities particularly in patients with convalescent or resolved COVID-19 infections should be interpreted with caution until more robust prospective clinical trials suggest otherwise.

Several small studies report similar findings between COVID-19-associated and nonviral COVID-19-related myocarditis.[62,63] A small study reported that acute mRNA vaccination-associated myocarditis can mimic acute viral myocarditis, both sharing similar CMR patterns. Evertz and colleagues[62] compared 10 acute mRNA vaccination-associated myocarditis and 10 acute viral myocarditis cases and reported that both groups had similar volumetric and functional parameters, lateral LV localization of LGE, and LGE extent. Similar findings were demonstrated by Haberka and colleagues[63] who reported that COVID-19-associated myocarditis and non–COVID-19-associated myocarditis share similarities in several ways. First, both groups had similar numbers of injured segments in the left ventricle, with most segments showing a minor (<25%) transmural extent of LGE. Second, both groups had similar volumetric and functional consequences with mild LVEF reduction, and a similar number of injured segments. Third, both groups had similar total LV LGE. There was, however, a higher rate of pericarditis in the COVID-19 group, suggesting that COVID-19 can cause perimyocardial injury specific for myocarditis and that it is important for clinicians to be aware of this complication. A case of acute COVID-19-related myocarditis and CMR findings discussed above are presented in **Fig. 3**.

FUTURE DIRECTIONS

Research studying new CMR imaging techniques, including strain analysis, feature tracking, texture analysis, and artificial intelligence are likely to improve the diagnostic and prognostic role of

CMR even further. For example, the addition of strain analysis to native T1 and T2 showed superior diagnostic accuracy compared with LLC alone. Additionally, strain analysis may replace LVEF as a useful biomarker for the diagnosis and prognostication of AM, especially in patients with preserved LVEF. Although results suggest these developments may offer superior diagnostic performance when compared with traditional biomarkers, large prospective trials are still needed to guide management of myocarditis patients effectively.[11,43]

Multiple studies continue to compare emerging diagnostic modalities for myocarditis diagnosis

with other well-established methods.[64–66] Meindl and colleagues[64] compared echocardiography with strain imaging and CMR with LGE. The study found that echocardiography using strain imaging had higher diagnostic accuracy and sensitivity than CMR using LGE in detecting myocarditis in patients with preserved systolic left ventricular function. Moreover, global and regional longitudinal strain provides important information on the mechanical function of the heart in patients with AM by quantifying the degree of myocardial dysfunction and determining if it is global or regional in nature. Furthermore, the study found that strain imaging was more sensitive than LGE

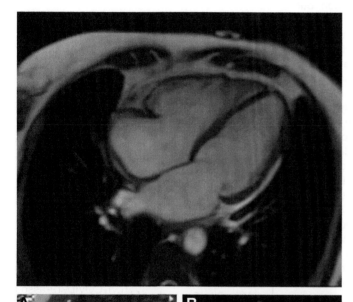

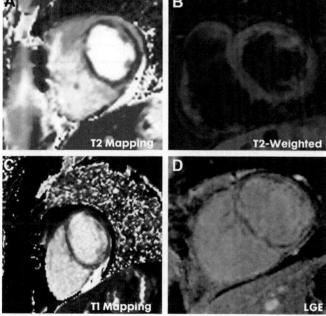

Fig. 3. CMR findings in a case of acute COVID-19 myocarditis. A 35-year-old man with chest pain due to suspected acute COVID-19 myocarditis received CMR, which showed acute interstitial edema on (*A*) increased value on T2-mapping (62 ms) and (*B*) T2-weighed-imaging with nonischemic myocardial injury based on (*C*) T1-mapping (increased 1365 ms, ECV 30%) and a (*D*) diffuse, patchy LGE pattern.

Table 2
Comparing the diagnostic utility of noninvasive imaging modalities for acute myocarditis

Diagnostic Modality	Diagnostic Accuracy (%)	Sensitivity (%)	Specificity (%)
Echocardiography (GLS)	93	78	93
CMR (Original LLC)	76	79	73
CMR (Updated LLC)	92	95	87

Note that the diagnostic accuracy, sensitivity, specificity values should apply to the specific population and diagnostic tests that was used to conduct each individual study and are not considered generalizable to myocarditis as a whole.

Abbreviations: (C)MR, cardiac magnetic resonance; CT, computed tomography; GLS, global longitudinal strain; LLC, Lake Louise Criteria; PET, positron emission tomography.

by CMR in detecting myocarditis in patients with preserved systolic left ventricular function but CMR with LGE was found to be more sensitive in detecting subclinical myocardial inflammation than strain analysis. In another study, Hsiao and colleagues[65] also reported that speckle tracking echocardiography (STE) can be a valuable tool in the diagnosis and management of AM. The study found that STE can accurately detect myocardial dysfunction in patients with AM and may be useful in monitoring disease progression and treatment response. Chen and colleagues[66] compared the diagnostic accuracy of CMR, PET/computed tomography (CT), and PET/MR in the detection of myocarditis and found that PET/MR had the highest diagnostic accuracy among the 3 imaging modalities, followed by CMR and then by PET/CT. Although results from these studies are promising, as seen in **Table 2**, larger, more robust clinical trials are required to provide additional guidance to management recommendations for myocarditis.

SUMMARY

Advancements in quantitative CMR has supplanted EMB for the diagnosis, risk stratification, and monitoring of clinically stable patients with acute viral myocarditis. Although CMR offers superior diagnostic accuracy, tissue characterization, and prognostication for these patients, EMB followed by immunohistochemistry and viral genome detection may be required to evaluate unstable or severely complicated AM and may become more useful as specific therapies targeting viral persistence or autoimmune-mediated inflammation become available. Although there is growing interest in studying COVID-19-associated CMR abnormalities and the application of new CMR imaging techniques to traditional evaluation, the evidence base supporting their use is limited and more robust, prospective clinical trials are required.

CLINICS CARE POINTS

- Initial diagnostic evaluation of suspected myocarditis includes history, physical, ECG, inflammatory and cardiac biomarkers, echocardiography, and CMR.[47]
- For stable patients with high suspicion for AM, CMR is recommended for diagnosis, myocardial tissue characterization, and differentiation of ischemic from nonischemic myocardial damage using LGE sequences but should be avoided in patients with a low-clinical suspicion.[11,47]
- Patients with myocarditis and symptomatic LV dysfunction should receive treatment according to heart failure guidelines.[47]
- Patients with DCM, NYHA class II-IV, and LVEF of 35% or lesser should receive primary prevention ICD placement.[18]
- After 3 to 6 months of initial evaluation, patients should receive a comprehensive reevaluation with laboratory and imaging studies to assess for resolution, complications (ie, VA, DCM), and safe return to sports.[50–52]

DISCLOSURES

The authors have no disclosures.

REFERENCES

1. Harding D, Chong MHA, Lahoti N, et al. Dilated cardiomyopathy and chronic cardiac inflammation: Pathogenesis, diagnosis and therapy. J Intern Med 2022. https://doi.org/10.1111/joim.13556.
2. Caforio ALP, Pankuweit S, Arbustini E, et al. Current state of knowledge on aetiology, diagnosis, management, and therapy of myocarditis: a position statement of the European Society of Cardiology Working Group on Myocardial and Pericardial Diseases. Eur Heart J 2013;34(33):2636–48.

3. Kindermann I, Barth C, Mahfoud F, et al. Update on myocarditis. J Am Coll Cardiol 2012;59(9):779–92.

4. Heymans S, Eriksson U, Lehtonen J, et al. The Quest for New Approaches in Myocarditis and Inflammatory Cardiomyopathy. J Am Coll Cardiol 2016; 68(21):2348–64.

5. Basso C. Myocarditis. N Engl J Med 2022;387(16): 1488–500.

6. Ammirati E, Frigerio M, Adler ED, et al. Management of Acute Myocarditis and Chronic Inflammatory Cardiomyopathy: An Expert Consensus Document. Circ Heart Fail 2020;13(11):E007405.

7. Baughman KL. Diagnosis of myocarditis death of Dallas criteria. Circulation 2006;113(4):593–5.

8. Bennett MK, Gilotra NA, Harrington C, et al. Evaluation of the role of endomyocardial biopsy in 851 patients with unexplained heart failure from 2000-2009. Circ Heart Fail 2013;6(4):676–84.

9. Singh V, Mendirichaga R, Savani GT, et al. Comparison of Utilization Trends, Indications, and Complications of Endomyocardial Biopsy in Native Versus Donor Hearts (from the Nationwide Inpatient Sample 2002 to 2014). Am J Cardiol 2018;121: 356–63.

10. Bozkurt B, Colvin M, Cook J, et al. Current Diagnostic and Treatment Strategies for Specific Dilated Cardiomyopathies: A Scientific Statement from the American Heart Association. Circulation 2016; 134(23):e579–646.

11. Ferreira VM, Schulz-Menger J, Holmvang G, et al. Cardiovascular Magnetic Resonance in Nonischemic Myocardial Inflammation: Expert Recommendations. J Am Coll Cardiol 2018;72(24):3158–76.

12. Lurz P, Eitel I, Adam J, et al. Diagnostic performance of CMR imaging compared with EMB in patients with suspected myocarditis. JACC Cardiovasc Imaging 2012;5(5):513–24.

13. Lurz P, Luecke C, Eitel I, et al. Comprehensive Cardiac Magnetic Resonance Imaging in Patients with Suspected Myocarditis the MyoRacer-Trial. J Am Coll Cardiol 2016;67(15):1800–11.

14. Shanbhag SM, Greve AM, Aspelund T, et al. Prevalence and prognosis of ischaemic and non-ischaemic myocardial fibrosis in older adults. Eur Heart J 2019. https://doi.org/10.1093/eurheartj/ehy876.

15. Kotanidis CP, Bazmpani MA, Haidich AB, et al. Diagnostic Accuracy of Cardiovascular Magnetic Resonance in Acute Myocarditis: A Systematic Review and Meta-Analysis. JACC Cardiovasc Imaging 2018;11(11):1583–90.

16. Lagan J, Schmitt M, Miller CA. Clinical applications of multi-parametric CMR in myocarditis and systemic inflammatory diseases. Int J Cardiovasc Imaging 2018;34:35–54.

17. Ammirati E, Cipriani M, Moro C, et al. Clinical presentation and outcome in a contemporary cohort of patients with acute myocarditis multicenter Lombardy registry. Circulation 2018;138(11):1088–99.

18. Ponikowski P, Voors AA, Anker SD, et al. ESC Guidelines for the diagnosis and treatment of acute and chronic heart failure. Eur Heart J 2016;37(27): 2129–2200m.

19. Cooper LT. Medical Progress Myocarditis. Lancet 2009;379(9817):738–47.

20. Gulati M, Levy PD, Mukherjee D, et al. AHA/ACC/ASE/CHEST/SAEM/SCCT/SCMR Guideline for the Evaluation and Diagnosis of Chest Pain: Executive Summary: A Report of the American College of Cardiology/American Heart Association Joint Committee on Clinical Practice Guidelines. Circulation 2021;144(22). https://doi.org/10.1161/CIR.0000000000001030.

21. Mahrholdt H, Wagner A, Deluigi CC, et al. Presentation, patterns of myocardial damage, and clinical course of viral myocarditis. Circulation 2006; 114(15):1581–90.

22. Aquaro GD, Perfetti M, Camastra G, et al. Cardiac MR With Late Gadolinium Enhancement in Acute Myocarditis With Preserved Systolic Function: IT-AMY Study. J Am Coll Cardiol 2017;70(16):1977–87.

23. Mavrogeni S, Manoussakis MN. Myocarditis as a Complication of Influenza A (H1N1): Evaluation Using Cardiovascular Magnetic Resonance Imaging. Hellenic J Cardiol 2010;51:379–80.

24. Friedrich MG, Sechtem U, Schulz-Menger J, et al. Cardiovascular Magnetic Resonance in Myocarditis: A JACC White Paper. J Am Coll Cardiol 2009;53(17): 1475–87.

25. Ferreira VM, Piechnik SK, Dall'armellina E, et al. Non-contrast T1-mapping detects acute myocardial edema with high diagnostic accuracy: a comparison to T2-weighted cardiovascular magnetic resonance. J Cardiovasc Magn Reson 2012;14:1.

26. Greulich S, Seitz A, Müller KAL, et al. Predictors of Mortality in Patients With Biopsy-Proven Viral Myocarditis: 10-Year Outcome Data. J AM Heart Assoc 2020. https://doi.org/10.1161/JAHA.119.015351.

27. Kindermann I, Kindermann M, Kandolf R, et al. Predictors of Outcome in Patients With Suspected Myocarditis. Circulation 2008. https://doi.org/10.1161/CIRCULATIONAHA.108.769489.

28. Grün S, Schumm J, Greulich S, et al. Long-Term Follow-Up of Biopsy-Proven Viral Myocarditis Predictors of Mortality and Incomplete Recovery. J AM Heart Assoc 2012. https://doi.org/10.1016/j.jacc.2012.01.007.

29. Georgiopoulos G, Figliozzi S, Sanguineti F, et al. Prognostic Impact of Late Gadolinium Enhancement by Cardiovascular Magnetic Resonance in Myocarditis: A Systematic Review and Meta-Analysis. Circ Cardiovasc Imaging 2021;14(1):E011492.

30. Luetkens JA, Homsi R, Dabir D, et al. Comprehensive Cardiac Magnetic Resonance for Short-Term

Follow-Up in Acute Myocarditis. J AM Heart Assoc 2016. https://doi.org/10.1161/JAHA.116.003603.

31. Donato Aquaro G, Habtemicael YG, Camastra G, et al. Prognostic Value of Repeating Cardiac Magnetic Resonance in Patients With Acute Myocarditis. J Am Coll Cardiol 2019. https://doi.org/10.1016/j.jacc.2019.08.1061.

32. Kim RJ, Fieno DS, Todd B, et al. Relationship of MRI Delayed Contrast Enhancement to Irreversible Injury, Infarct Age, and Contractile Function. Circulation 1999;100. Available at: http://www.circulationaha.org.

33. Spieker M, Haberkorn S, Gastl M, et al. Abnormal T2 mapping cardiovascular magnetic resonance correlates with adverse clinical outcome in patients with suspected acute myocarditis. J Cardiovasc Magn Reson 2017. https://doi.org/10.1186/s12968-017-0350-x.

34. Muser D, Nucifora G, Pieroni M, et al. Prognostic Value of Nonischemic Ringlike Left Ventricular Scar in Patients With Apparently Idiopathic Nonsustained Ventricular Arrhythmias. Circulation 2021;143(14):1359–73.

35. Chen W, Qian W, Zhang X, et al. Ring-like late gadolinium enhancement for predicting ventricular tachyarrhythmias in non-ischaemic dilated cardiomyopathy. Eur Heart J Cardiovasc Imaging 2021. https://doi.org/10.1093/ehjci/jeab117.

36. Stiermaier T, Föhrenbach F, Klingel K, et al. Biventricular endomyocardial biopsy in patients with suspected myocarditis: Feasibility, complication rate and additional diagnostic value. Int J Cardiol 2016. https://doi.org/10.1016/j.ijcard.2016.12.103.

37. Yilmaz A, Kindermann I, Kindermann M, et al. Comparative evaluation of left and right ventricular endomyocardial biopsy: Differences in complication rate and diagnostic performance. Circulation 2010;122(9):900–9.

38. Lauer B, Niederau C, Kühl U, et al. Cardiac Troponin T in Patients With Clinically Suspected Myocarditis. J Am Coll Cardiol 1997;30:1354–63.

39. Thygesen K, Alpert JS, Jaffe AS, et al. Fourth Universal Definition of Myocardial Infarction (2018). Circulation 2018;138(20):e618–51.

40. Smith SC, Ladenson JH, Mason JW, et al. Elevations of cardiac troponin I associated with myocarditis: Experimental and clinical correlates. Circulation 1997;95(1):163–8.

41. Morgera T, di Lenarda A, Dreas L, et al. Electrocardiography of myocarditis revisited: clinical and prognostic significance of electrocardiographic changes. Am Heart J 1992;124(2):455–67.

42. Ammann P, Naegeli B, Schuiki E, et al. independent of cardiac enzyme release. Int J Cardiol 2003;89:217–22.

43. Eichhorn C, Greulich S, Bucciarelli-Ducci C, et al. Multiparametric Cardiovascular Magnetic Resonance Approach in Diagnosing, Monitoring, and Prognostication of Myocarditis. JACC Cardiovasc Imaging 2022;15(7):1325–38.

44. Gräni C, Bière Loïc, Christian Eichhorn, et al. Incremental value of extracellular volume assessment by cardiovascular magnetic resonance imaging in risk stratifying patients with suspected myocarditis. Int J Cardiovasc Imaging 2019;35:1067–78.

45. Kuethe F, Franz M, Jung C, et al. Outcome predictors in dilated cardiomyopathy or myocarditis. Eur J Clin Invest 2017;47(7):513–23.

46. Chopra H, Arangalage D, Bouleti C, et al. Prognostic value of the infarct-and non-infarct like patterns and cardiovascular magnetic resonance parameters on long-term outcome of patients after acute myocarditis. Int J Cardiol 2016. https://doi.org/10.1016/j.ijcard.2016.03.004.

47. McDonagh TA, Metra M, Adamo M, et al. ESC Guidelines for the diagnosis and treatment of acute and chronic heart failureDeveloped by the Task Force for the diagnosis and treatment of acute and chronic heart failure of the European Society of Cardiology (ESC) With the special contribution of the Heart Failure Association (HFA) of the ESC. Eur Heart J 2021;42(36):3599–726.

48. Halliday BP, Cleland JGF, Goldberger JJ, et al. Personalizing Risk Stratification for Sudden Death in Dilated Cardiomyopathy: The Past, Present, and Future. Circulation 2017;136(2):215–31.

49. Yancy CW, Jessup M, Bozkurt B, et al. ACCF/AHA guideline for the management of heart failure: A report of the american college of cardiology foundation/american heart association task force on practice guidelines. Circulation 2013;128(16). https://doi.org/10.1161/CIR.0B013E31829E8776/FORMAT/EPUB.

50. Klem I, Klein M, Khan M, et al. Relationship of LVEF and Myocardial Scar to Long-Term Mortality Risk and Mode of Death in Patients with Nonischemic Cardiomyopathy. Circulation 2021;143(14):1343–58.

51. Pelliccia A, Corrado D, Bjärnstad HH, et al. Recommendations for participation in competitive sport and leisure-time physical activity in individuals with cardiomyopathies, myocarditis and pericarditis. Eur J Prev Cardiol 2006;13(6):876–85.

52. Maron BJ, Udelson JE, Bonow RO, et al. Eligibility and Disqualification Recommendations for Competitive Athletes with Cardiovascular Abnormalities: Task Force 3: Hypertrophic Cardiomyopathy, Arrhythmogenic Right Ventricular Cardiomyopathy and Other Cardiomyopathies, and Myocarditis: A Scientific Statement from the American Heart Association and American College of Cardiology. Circulation 2015;132(22):e273–80.

53. D'Ascenzi F, Solari M, Corrado D, et al. Diagnostic Differentiation Between Arrhythmogenic Cardiomyopathy and Athlete's Heart by Using Imaging. JACC Cardiovasc Imaging 2018;11(9):1327–39.

54. Zorzi A, Marra MP, Rigato I, et al. Nonischemic left ventricular scar as a substrate of life-threatening ventricular arrhythmias and sudden cardiac death in competitive athletes. Circ Arrhythm Electrophysiol 2016;9(7). https://doi.org/10.1161/CIRCEP.116.004229/FORMAT/EPUB.

55. Anzini M, Merlo M, Sabbadini G, et al. Long-term evolution and prognostic stratification of biopsy-proven active myocarditis. Circulation 2013;128(22):2384–94.

56. Bohm P, Rgen Scharhag J, Meyer T. European society of cardiology ® Original scientific paper Data from a nationwide registry on sports-related sudden cardiac deaths in Germany. Eur J Prev Cardiol 2016. https://doi.org/10.1177/2047487315594087.

57. Tschöpe C, Ammirati E, Bozkurt B, et al. Myocarditis and inflammatory cardiomyopathy: current evidence and future directions. Nat Rev Cardiol 2021. https://doi.org/10.1038/s41569-020-00435-x.

58. Dweck MR, Bularga A, Hahn RT, et al. Global evaluation of echocardiography in patients with COVID-19. Eur Heart J Cardiol imagine 2020. https://doi.org/10.1093/ehjci/jeaa178.

59. Agricola E, Beneduce A, Esposito A, et al. Heart and Lung Multimodality Imaging in COVID-19. JACC Cardiovasc Imaging 2020;13(8):1792–808.

60. Pontone G, Baggiano A, Conte E, et al. Quadruple Rule-Out" With Computed Tomography in a COVID-19 Patient With Equivocal Acute Coronary Syndrome Presentation. JACC Cardiovasc Imaging 2020;13(8):1854–6.

61. Wilson M, O'Hanlon R, Prasad S, et al. Diverse patterns of myocardial fibrosis in lifelong, veteran endurance athletes. J Appl Physiol 2011;110(6):1622.

62. Evertz R, Schulz A, Lange T, et al. Cardiovascular magnetic resonance imaging patterns of acute COVID-19 mRNA vaccine-associated myocarditis in young male patients: A first single-center experience. Front Cardiovasc Med 2022;9:2217. https://doi.org/10.3389/FCVM.2022.965512/BIBTEX.

63. Haberka M, Rajewska-Tabor J, Wojtowicz D, et al. Perimyocardial Injury Specific for SARS-CoV-2-Induced Myocarditis in Comparison With Non-COVID-19 Myocarditis: A Multicenter CMR Study. JACC Cardiovasc Imaging 2022;15(4):705–7.

64. Meindl C, Paulus Michael, Poschenrieder F, et al. Patients with acute myocarditis and preserved systolic left ventricular function: comparison of global and regional longitudinal strain imaging by echocardiography with quantification of late gadolinium enhancement by CMR Keywords Myocarditis · CMR · Speckle tracking · Regional longitudinal strain. Clin Res Cardiol 2021;110:1792–800.

65. Hsiao JF, Koshino Y, Bonnichsen CR, et al. Speckle tracking echocardiography in acute myocarditis. Int J Cardiovasc Imaging 2013. https://doi.org/10.1007/s10554-012-0085-6.

66. Chen W, Jeudy J. Assessment of Myocarditis: Cardiac MR, PET/CT, or PET/MR? Curr Cardiol Rep 2019;21(8):1–10.

Heart Failure Preserved Ejection Fraction in Women: Insights Learned from Imaging

Edoardo Sciatti, MD[a], Michela Giovanna Coccia, MD[b],
Roberta Magnano, MD[c], Gupta Aakash, MD[d], Raul Limonta, MD[e],
Brian Diep, MD[d], Giulio Balestrieri, MD[a], Salvatore D'Isa, MD[a],
Dmitry Abramov, MD[d], Purvi Parwani, MBBS, MPH[d],
Emilia D'Elia, MD, PhD, FESC[a],*

KEYWORDS

- Heart failure preserved ejection fraction • Women • Sex differences • Imaging technique

KEY POINTS

- There is growing evidence for sex-specific features in patients with heart failure with preserved ejection fraction (HFpEF), including differences in characteristics between men and women which are apparent at imaging techniques.
- Differences in cardiac physiology, cardiovascular risk factors, immune system, and hormonal balance lead to different phenotypes of HFpEF according to gender, and imaging must become more tailored to these concepts and clinical observations.
- A multi-modality imaging approach is recommended to identify specific forms of disease and to better identify the origin of diastolic dysfunction, which could reach various degrees of severity according, also, to gender.
- Sex-related differences in echo parameters at rest and under stress, left and right chambers strain, exercise stress test, and cardiac magnetic resonance can be detected, described, and used to better phenotype HFpEF.

INTRODUCTION

Heart failure with preserved ejection fraction (HFpEF) is a complex clinical syndrome in which sex-specific features due to anatomical, physiological, and hormonal characteristics contribute to different clinical phenotypes.[1] Women are more subjected to develop HFpEF as they experience more concentric left ventricle hypertrophy, more atrial, ventricular, and arterial stiffness, and less ventricular dilation compared to men, all of which predisposes to higher degree of diastolic dysfunction (DD).[2] Imaging is of utmost importance in detecting these sex differences, and a multi-modality approach in HFpEF should be encouraged, as it could provide precious insights of the disease, with different characterizations between women and men.

To this regard, this review focuses on the most common and pathognomonic HFpEF differences according to sex detected by imaging. With growing evidence for unique mechanisms,

Note: Sex refers to "the different biological and physiological characteristics of males and females, such as reproductive organs, chromosomes, hormones, etc." Gender refers to "the socially constructed characteristics of women and men–such as norms, roles and relationships of and between groups of women and men. In this article term "women" and "female" even though used interchangeably, refer to female.

[a] Cardiology Unit, Hospital Papa Giovanni XXIII, Bergamo, Italy; [b] Cardiology Unit, Voghera Hospital, ASST Pavia, Voghera, Italy; [c] Cardiology Unit, Hospital Santo Spirito, Pescara, Italy; [d] Division of Cardiology, Department of Medicine, Loma Linda University Health, Loma Linda, CA, USA; [e] School of Medicine and Surgery, Milano Bicocca University, Milano, Italy
* Corresponding author. Cardiovascular Department, Hospital Papa Giovanni XXIII, Piazza OMS 1, Bergamo, Italy.
E-mail address: edelia@asst-pg23.it

pathophysiology, and manifestations involved in women with HFpEF, the role of imaging must become more tailored as well. Here, we review the latest evidence on how various imaging modalities are being utilized and analyzed to provide more individualized evaluation in women.

HEART FAILURE WITH PRESERVED EJECTION FRACTION: DEFINITION AND DIAGNOSIS

Heart failure with preserved ejection fraction (HFpEF) is defined, in terms of hemodynamics, by the presence of elevated left ventricular (LV) filling pressure, either at rest or during exercise, in the setting of a normal left ventricular ejection fraction (LVEF) of greater than or equal to 50%.[3] Given that LV filling occurs during diastole, HFpEF is a disease of DD.[4] The main signs of HFpEF is congestion, such as jugular vein distension, orthopnea, edema, and third heart sound, along with symptoms including breathlessness, fatigue, and paroxysmal nocturnal dyspnea. The etiology of HFpEF is multifactorial-it typically evolves from a combination of risk factors and comorbidities that affect the myocardium via mechanisms including myocyte hypertrophy, interstitial fibrosis, inflammation, and oxidative stress. These processes lead to abnormal diastolic relaxation, increased end-diastolic stiffness, reduced LV compliance, and, in turn, left atrial and ventricular dysfunction.[5]

HFpEF can be clinically diagnosed by the presence of symptoms typical for HF with evidence of cardiac structural and/or functional abnormalities consistent with LV diastolic dysfunction or raised LV filling pressures.[6] Outside of invasive hemodynamic studies, no single measure is sensitive or specific enough to confirm the presence of HFpEF, so a constellation of suggestive signs in the patient's history, laboratory testing, electrocardiography, echocardiography, or advanced imaging is required. Characteristic findings include laboratory testing demonstrating elevated natriuretic peptides (NPs) and echocardiography demonstrating LV hypertrophy, abnormal velocity across the mitral valve (such as increased E/e' ratio), elevated pulmonary artery pressure (derived from tricuspid regurgitation velocity) and increased left atrial volume.[7] The Heart Failure Association (HFA) of the European Society of Cardiology (ESC) has created a scoring system to diagnose HFpEF using these non-invasive measures.[8] The standard for HFpEF, involves left and right heart catheterization for hemodynamic monitoring at rest and with exercise, although invasive or complex evaluation many be challenging in the community setting.[9] HFpEF is confirmed if LV end-diastolic pressure (LVEDP) is greater than 16 mm Hg or pulmonary capillary wedge pressure (PCWP) is greater than 15 mm Hg at rest, or PCWP is greater than 25 mm Hg during exercise (**Fig. 1**). To then determine etiology, stress tests and/or more-detailed imaging such as cardiac magnetic resonance (CMR) can be used.[10]

Given the varying contributing factors, etiologies, and pathophysiological expressions of HFpEF, newer perspectives label HFpEF as a complex clinical syndrome rather than a single diagnosis, and, in this framework, a more specific iconographic approach considering sex-specific features of HFpEF will prompt more individualized and effective management.

GENDER: A HEART FAILURE WITH PRESERVED EJECTION FRACTION RISK FACTOR

Women have unique anatomical and physiological features that should be considered during diagnostic and management assessment of suspected HFpEF.

While the prevalence of HF, in general, is similar in men and women, women experience a higher rate of HFpEF relative to HFrEF (Odds ratio = 2.0 in women vs. 0.72 in men).[11]

There are several reasons to explain this imbalance. Some risk factors for HFpEF exhibit a higher prevalence in women compared to men, such as obesity (4 to 29% higher in women) and anemia. Parity, a risk factor exclusive to women, is also associated with long-term adverse cardiac remodeling and dysfunction, in part due to the significant increase in cardiac output during pregnancy.[12,13] Some risk factors, though exhibiting a similar prevalence between sexes, disproportionately increase the risk of HFpEF in women compared to men, such as increased age, hypertension, diabetes, and smoking.[14–16] For example, studies have found that in response to increasing age and hypertension, women experience more concentric LV remodeling, more ventricular and arterial stiffness, and less ventricular dilation compared to men, which predisposes women to developing diastolic dysfunction.[17,18] The pathophysiology for this disparity may be partly explained by the baseline differences in women's normal cardiac physiology, the interaction of these risk factors with estrogen, a hormone that is cardio-protective for women, and/or the unique characteristics of women's immune system.[19,20]

The immune system and inflammation play a pivotal role in the development of HFpEF, and given that women have stronger immune responses than men, these chronic conditions may

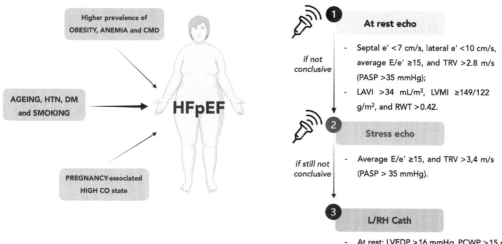

Fig. 1. Epidemiology, Risk Factors, and Diagnosis of Heart Failure with Preserved Ejection Fraction (HFpEF). HFpEF has a higher incidence in women than in men and appears to be associated with a greater prevalence of specific risk factors such as obesity, coronary microvascular disease, and anemia. Additionally, in women, the effect of aging, cigarette smoking, hypertension, and diabetes mellitus appears to have a greater effect on ventricular remodeling than in men (*thick arrow*). The presence of all these factors seems to justify the higher incidence of diastolic dysfunction and subsequently HFpEF in women. Furthermore, women have exceptional occurrence of pregnancy, which imposes an increased workload on the left ventricle related to the high output state throughout the entire gestation period, and parity is proportional to the future extent of diastolic dysfunction. In both women and men, the diagnosis requires the demonstration of the morpho-functional alterations related to HFpEF. All patients undergo resting echocardiography, followed by stress echocardiography in case of uncertainty, and finally left and right heart catheterization, which can reveal, in a progressively invasive manner, the increase in ventricular filling pressures during physical exertion. CMD, coronary microvascular disease; CO, cardiac output; DM, diabetes mellitus; HTN, hypertension; LAVI, left atrium volume index; LVEDP, left ventricular end-diastolic pressure; LVMI, left ventricle mass index; PASP, pulmonary artery pressure systolic pressure; PCWP, pulmonary capillary wedge pressure; RWT, relative wall thickness; TRV, tricuspid regurgitation velocity.

cause a greater impact on cardiac dysfunction in women compared to men.[21]

At rest, women have higher mitral inflow velocity to diastolic mitral annular velocity at early filling (E/e′) ratio with a relatively higher ejection fraction and smaller ventricular dimension.[22] With a history of increased parity, women with HFpEF experience even more severe dysfunction; one study found that a history of three or more births was associated with increased PCWP, right atrial pressure, pulmonary vascular resistance, and lower LVEF, compared to female patients with HFpEF with less than three births[23] (**Fig. 2**).

MULTIMODALITY IMAGING DIAGNOSIS OF HEART FAILURE WITH PRESERVED EJECTION FRACTION IN WOMEN

Given the shift toward considering HFpEF a clinical syndrome with pathophysiology that varies between sexes, a multi-modality imaging approach is recommended to identify specific forms of disease and to better identify the origin of structural and functional cardiac abnormalities.[24] Relevant imaging modalities include echocardiography, coronary angiography, computed tomography (CT), cardiac magnetic resonance (CMR), positron emission tomography (PET), single photon emission computed tomography (SPECT), cardiac scintigraphy, right and left heart catheterization, and stress or exercise imaging[25] (**Fig. 3**).

Myocardial Structure and Function

Fundamental underlying sex differences in myocardial structure and function detected by echocardiography have been documented in literature.[26] In general, women display a higher LVEF than men, this difference becoming more pronounced with age. Indeed, a substantial decrease in LV end-systolic volume in aging women accounts for a concomitant increase in LVEF.[27] Noteworthy, sex differences exist even within normal cardiac chambers dimensions, with women presenting lower left and right chambers volumes as well as LV mass, even after correcting

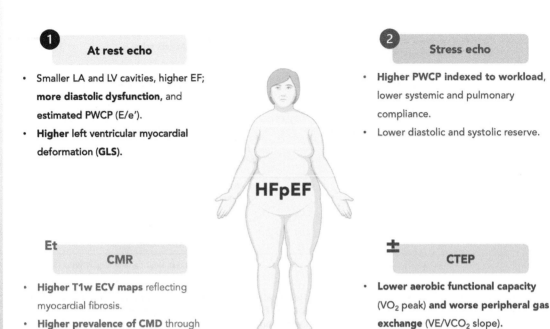

1 **At rest echo**

- Smaller LA and LV cavities, higher EF; **more diastolic dysfunction,** and estimated PWCP (E/e').
- **Higher** left ventricular myocardial deformation (**GLS**).

2 **Stress echo**

- **Higher PWCP indexed to workload,** lower systemic and pulmonary compliance.
- Lower diastolic and systolic reserve.

Et **CMR**

- **Higher T1w ECV maps** reflecting myocardial fibrosis.
- **Higher prevalence of CMD** through MPRi and MPR during stress.

± **CTEP**

- **Lower aerobic functional capacity** (VO$_2$ peak) **and worse peripheral gas exchange** (VE/VCO$_2$ slope).

HFpEF

Fig. 2. Non-invasive imaging in Women: sex-specific findings. Resting echocardiography serves as the cornerstone for the diagnosis of heart failure with preserved ejection fraction (HFpEF) owing to its ability to provide a comprehensive assessment of cardiac morphology and function. Notably, women with HFpEF exhibit smaller atrial and ventricular cavities, a phenomenon that corresponds to a compensatory increase in ejection fraction. Additionally, female myocardium displays an exaggerated response to afterload, leading to concentric hypertrophy, which ultimately predisposes to both pronounced, early diastolic dysfunction and altered global longitudinal strain of the left ventricle. In cases of diagnostic uncertainty, exercise echocardiography may unmask occult HFpEF by revealing higher ventricular filling pressures in women during specific workloads compared to men. Such differences could potentially reflect the reduced systolic and diastolic reserve of female patients. These morpho-functional findings are further supported by the results of cardiopulmonary exercise testing, which suggests that women experience a greater reduction in functional capacity despite displaying the characteristic dyspnea and exercise intolerance associated with HFpEF. Finally, cardiac magnetic resonance imaging (CMRI) can aid in the identification of the etiology of heart failure, which often involves microvascular coronary disease. Specifically, CMRI may demonstrate a high prevalence of semi-quantitative (MPRi) and quantitative (MPR) myocardial perfusion defects during stress acquisitions. Additionally, T1-weighted images can identify and quantify fibrosis, which appears to be more prevalent in women and may serve as a predictor of prognosis. CMD, coronary microvascular dysfunction; CMR, cardiac magnetic resonance; CPET, cardiopulmonary exercise test; DASI, duke activity status index; ECV, extracellular volume; EF, ejection fraction; Et, etiology; GLS, left ventricle global longitudinal strain; LA, left atrium; LV LV, left ventricle; MPR, myocardial perfusion reserve; MPRi, myocardial perfusion reserve index; PWCP, pulmonary wedge capillary pressure.

for body surface area.[28] In the PARAMOUNT study, women displayed greater cardiac functional abnormalities than men, with a greater degree of LV hypertrophy in response to hypertension and obesity compared to men.[2] Moreover, women have been shown to display a steeper increase of LV mass with aging, it being understood that there are different LV mass cut-offs in women compared to men LV mass index > 95 g/m2 in women and >115 g/m2 in men.[29] In several echocardiographic study performed in this setting, HFpEF women were more likely to have concentric LV remodeling with smaller LV diameters and higher LVEF, together with a more pronounced

DD, a higher prevalence of CMD, and greater degree of arterial stiffness.[30–33] Compared to men, women display a higher peak A wave velocity, consequently a lower E/A ratio, a higher LV systolic stiffness, and a greater degree of LV reserve impairment, the latter been ascribed a central role in HFpEF pathophysiology.[34,35]

CMR imaging is an expanding method that has become part of clinical practice, answering numerous clinical questions in patients with HF without the use of ionizing radiation, integrating and complementing the echocardiographic study.[36] Similar to echocardiographic reference ranges, reference ranges of cardiac structures

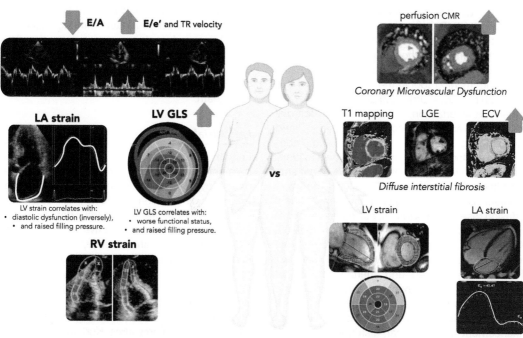

Fig. 3. The female heart differs partly from that of males. Firstly, it exhibits smaller atrial and ventricular cavities, which, in the case of diastolic dysfunction, accounts for the disproportionate increase in atrial contribution (A) compared to early rapid filling (E) and consequently results in more pronounced elevations in tele-diastolic pressures (E/e') assessed via echocardiography. Furthermore, the geometric configuration of the female left ventricle also justifies higher values of global longitudinal strain (GLS) compared to males, serving as an indirect parameter of increased filling pressures (similarly to atrial strain) and impaired functional capacity. The investigation of right ventricular (RV) geometry and, notably, function has demonstrated prognostic implications in patients with heart failure with preserved ejection fraction (HFpEF). Left ventricle (LV) GLS and LA strain are also assessed using cardiac magnetic resonance imaging (CMR), which, moreover, proves useful in identifying a specific etiology (such as coronary microvascular dysfunction) and quantifying intramyocardial fibrosis. CMR, cardiac magnetic resonance; ECV, extra-cellular volume; GLS, global longitudinal strain; LA, left atrium; LGE, late gadolinium enhancement; LV, left ventricle; RV, right ventricle.

including myocardial mass and chamber volumes by MRI are sex specific.[37,38] LV volumes, both absolute and indexed, and mass are smaller in women than men, while EF is equal or greater.[38–41]

Myocardial Fibrosis

HFpEF is predominantly associated with many comorbidities and risk factors related to myocyte (titin changes), interstitial (extracellular matrix and inflammation with or within fibrosis), microvascular and metabolic abnormalities[42,43] Coronary microvascular rarefaction on CMR has been shown to be one of the key histological features in an autopsy study of patients with HFpEF and was associated with increased myocardial fibrosis.[44] Diffuse myocardial fibrosis assessed by extracellular volume (ECV) characterizes a vulnerable interstitium correlated with LV stiffness measured invasively by pressure-volume loop and has been associated with disease severity and prognosis in HFpEF. In a recent large study, ECV was

elevated in asymptomatic patients at risk for HFpEF, moreover it was associated with increased NPs, even in the absence of signs or symptoms of HF.[45,46] Diffuse myocardial fibrosis assessed by ECV characterizes a vulnerable interstitium correlated with LV stiffness measured invasively by pressure-volume loop, and has been associated with disease severity and prognosis in HFpEF. According to the several CMR studies in literature, women younger than 45 years have a higher T1 mapping value than men, furthermore there is a trend towards a lower native T1 mapping value with increasing age (about 20 ms more for women younger than 45 years than for women older than 45 years).[47] Even according to MESA (Multi-Ethnic Study of Atherosclerosis) data, with higher risk prevalence, a higher ECV is observed in women.[48]

Coronary Vasculature

Women have a much higher prevalence of ischemia with non-obstructive coronary arteries

(INOCA)[49] as well as coronary microvascular dysfunction (CMD),[50,51] which are closely linked risk factors for HFpEF, and therefore should be given attention when choosing and analyzing imaging tests for ischemic evaluation. CMR is a key diagnostic imaging tool in the assessment of patients with MINOCA, providing detailed myocardial tissue characterization, location of myocardial inflammation/edema, scarring/fibrosis, and discriminating between ischemic and non-ischemic etiologies. CMR has been shown to identify the underlying etiology in up to 87% of patients with MINOCA.[52] Exercise CMRi allows the measurement of the semi-quantitative myocardial perfusion reserve index (MPRI, cut-off value < 1.84) and quantitative myocardial perfusion reserve (MPR, cut-off value < 2.19), which have been shown to have high sensitivity and specificity for CMD both in women and men. One-third of women with INOCA (non-obstructive ischemic coronary artery disease) do not have a diagnosis of previous MI, but about 8% can have late enhancement with atypical distribution[53] which can contribute to diastolic dysfunction and eventually HFpEF. Interestingly, abnormal perfusion noted on stress CMR is likely to be related also to microvascular dysfunction.[54] A recent study demonstrates that CMR can predict prognosis in patients with INOCA, independent of sex.[55]

Global Longitudinal Strain

Assessment of myocardial deformation using 2D speckle-tracking echocardiography for the measurement of global longitudinal strain (GLS) has emerged as a more sensitive and objective modality than LVEF alone to quantify LV contractile performance and may represent a useful tool to characterize HFpEF population,[56,57] showing higher cut-off of LV GLS in women compared to men.[58] The difference in LV mass between men and women is attributed to the smaller hearts of women, even when indexed to body size, resulting in smaller LV volumes and lower LV mass.[59] To compensate for smaller cavity size, women have a slightly higher LVEF, and a consequently higher GLS. Greater longitudinal deformation was observed in women compared to men, with similar circumferential deformation persisting across a broad age variability.[60] Additionally, there is less cardiomyocyte loss in women during a lifespan, and it has been proposed that women are less susceptible to decreases in contractility when afterload increases, as compared to men.[61] Studies investigating surrogate markers of HFpEF severity in outpatient clinical setting found that impaired regional LV GLS is associated with worse

scores on the Duke Activity Status Index, while abnormal LV GLS correlated with increased NPs, and decreased peak oxygen consumption (VO2) at cardiopulmonary exercise test.[62] Moreover, GLS has been shown to be a potential predictor of HF-related hospitalizations and cardiovascular (CV) death.[63,64]

Left Atrial Strain

Left atrial longitudinal strain, an angle-independent parameter derived from speckle-tracking echocardiography, is a relatively novel method to assess the reservoir function of the LA. LA strain (LAs) has been documented as an important prognostic parameter, underlying the active role of LA in the pathophysiology of the disease,[65] as it is significantly linked to DD severity.[66–68] LAs were also found to be more sensitive than LAVI in detecting LA impairment in HFpEF, as it inversely correlates with LV DD severity and it is superior to LA ejection fraction, LAVI, or E/e′ in predicting the presence of elevated LV filling pressures. Kurt and colleagues[69] showed that LA strain could accurately discriminated HFpEF from hypertensive patients, similarly, Obokata and colleagues[70] found that LAs could distinguish HFpEF from the hypertension control group at rest. No specific differences in LAs among sex were detected in a meta-analysis of multiple databases of 2 clinical trials and 12 observational studies, comprising 1974 patients with HFpEF and 751 healthy controls.[71]

Magnetic resonance imaging allows a comprehensive study of the function and size of the LA, in particular LAVI and LAs. Absolute left atrial volume is smaller in women than men, while indexed left atrial volume and emptying fraction are similar between sexes.[38]

Altered atrial function, frequently related to altered LV mechanic, is an early predictor of the progression of the disease in symptomatic HFpEF.[72] CMRi studies in patients with HFpEF have shown that conduit is an early precursor of atrial remodeling. Reservoir and conduit are reduced in patients with HFpEF and conduit is the strongest predictor of exercise intolerance.[73] Strain values are comparable between genders, while LA booster pump and conduit function parameters change significantly with age in both sex.[74] Feature tracking at advanced CMR (CMR-FT) assess LA function through strain (distinguishing three phases of conduit, reservoir, and pump) overcoming the limitations of echocardiography (spatial resolution and reproducibility). Various studies did not show a difference between gender composition and LA assessment of reservoir, conduit, and contractile strain.[74–76]

Right Ventricular Structure and Function

Right ventricular (RV) function is a major determinant of prognosis and adverse outcomes in patients with HFpEF.[77] Assessment of RV function can be performed by multiple echo parameters, including tricuspid annular plane systolic excursion (TAPSE), systolic velocity of tricuspid annulus (S′), fractional area change, RV myocardial performance (Tei index), RV dP/dt, RVEF and RV strain.[78,79] Transthoracic echo also enables the measurement of pulmonary artery systolic pressure (PASP): pulmonary arterial hypertension (PAH) is more common in women, particularly due to autoimmune disease as systemic sclerosis.[80–83] The contribution of dynamic RV-pulmonary arterial (RV-PA) coupling between sex and its impact on peak exercise capacity (VO2) in HFpEF is not known. In an interesting study investigating the differential effects of sex on RV-PA coupling during maximum incremental exercise in patients with HFpEF, male patients were more compromised regarding dynamic RV-PA uncoupling and reduced peak VO2 compared with female. Female patients, instead, had preserved RV-PA coupling during exercise and better peak exercise VO2 compared with male.[84]

RV volumes indexed for BSA are larger in men than women, and abnormalities of RV by CMRi have been found to be independently associated with outcome and clinical status in HFpEF.[85,86] Using CMR, both absolute and indexed RV volumes are smaller in women compared to men, while RV ejection fraction is greater or equal in women compared to men.[38–41]

Pulmonary arterial hypertension (PAH) is a rare disease with higher mortality due to pre-capillary pulmonary hypertension and consequent RV failure.[87] It is more common in women, typically regarding PAH secondary to systemic sclerosis.[88] CMR studies have shown that women with PAH have better RV function than men at baseline.[89] CMR has unique capabilities to evaluate RV structure and function as well as septal abnormalities in patients with PAH,[90] and can be used to predict prognosis.[91,92] Myocardial fibrosis at the RV insertions on the interventricular septum found by LGE CMR is a typical feature in PH.[93] Of note, the presence of LGE is related to the degree of RV dysfunction, the severity of PH,[94] and poorer clinical outcomes in PAH.[92] In addition, women show greater improvement in RV ejection fraction with PAH specific drugs compared to men.[95] The EURO-MR Study suggested that CMR could be used to assess clinical benefit of PAH-targeted medical therapy, where the improvement of RV and LV function and volumes was associated with patient survival.[96]

DIFFERENT IMAGING TECHNIQUES UNDER STRESS TO EXPLORE WOMEN CAPACITY IN HEART FAILURE WITH PRESERVED EJECTION FRACTION

In HFpEF, women display cardiometabolic profiles and exercise hemodynamic parameters significantly different compared to men.[97,98] During exercise stress test women with HFpEF were found to have, on average, higher PCWP indexed to workload, lower pulmonary and systemic arterial compliance, and a greater rise in lactate. Compared to men, they display higher mitral inflow velocity to diastolic mitral annular velocity at early filling ratios at rest and peak exercise, along with a higher LVEF and smaller ventricular dimensions.[99,100] One of the more specific stresses testing to perform diagnosis of HFpEF is cardiopulmonary exercise testing (CPET). It provides information on exercise capacity, gas exchange efficiency, and cardiovascular and respiratory function during exercise. One of the main parameters measured during CPET is peak oxygen consumption (VO2 peak), which is a marker of overall cardiorespiratory fitness or aerobic fitness. Another marker is VE/VCO2 slope, which is a measure of gas exchange efficiency during exercise. A higher VE/VCO2 slope indicates worse gas exchange efficiency during exercise, which can be an early marker for cardiovascular dysfunction.[101]

Rozenbaum and colleagues[102] investigated sex differences in CPET parameters in patients with HFpEF and found that women had lower VO2peak, VO2 at the ventilatory threshold, and anaerobic threshold as well as a higher VE/VCO2 slope than men. These findings suggest that women with HFpEF may have worse exercise capacity and gas exchange efficiency than men.

In another study, obesity was found to be more strongly associated with reduced VO2 peak and impaired diastolic function in women than in men with HFpEF. Diastolic function was found to be worse in obese women compared to obese men.[103] Pregnancy and parity also play a role in exercise physiology in women with HFpEF. One study found that higher parity (described as >3 pregnancies) was associated with lower VO2peak and worse diastolic function, suggesting that higher parity may be a risk factor for worse exercise capacity and cardiovascular function in HFpEF women.[18] Honigberg and colleagues investigated sex differences in exercise capacity and quality of life in patients with HFpEF. The study analyzed data from two randomized controlled trials and found that women had lower VO2 peak and lower six-minute walk distance (6MWD) compared to men.[104] In that study, women did not demonstrate an association between 6MWD and quality of life, unlike the positive association noted in men, which suggests that additional exercise metrics may be needed to better quantify the quality of life in women with HFpEF. Taken together, these studies suggest that sex-related differences in CPET parameters are an important consideration in the management of patients with HFpEF. Future studies should continue to explore the sex-specific differences in CPET parameters and exercise stress test echo parameters and their implications for the management of HFpEF.

DIFFERENTIAL DIAGNOSIS OF HEART FAILURE WITH PRESERVED EJECTION FRACTION ON CARDIAC MAGNETIC RESONANCE

In addition to above-mentioned imaging parameters, CMR can be useful in detecting various cardiovascular pathologies that are responsible for myocardial structural changes that lead to DD.[105] Cardiac amyloidosis is one such pathology, an infiltrative cardiomyopathy, principally related to immunoglobulin light chains in AL form and transthyretin protein in ATTR one and more frequent in male than female.[106] Early diagnosis is pivotal to start specific treatments since survival is poor if untreated.[107,108] Echocardiography is an important tool to raise suspicion against the presence of cardiac amyloidosis.[109] In the context of LV hypertrophy, pericardial and/or pleural effusions, RV hypertrophy, thick valves, and thick interatrial septum, small LV cavity size with low stroke volume, and valve thickening can be present in patients with cardiac amyloidosis.[110] In advanced forms restrictive LV filling pattern can be found. Finally, amyloid infiltration impairs GLS characteristically with the apical sparing of the LV apex and severely reduced contractile function of the atrial myocardium.[111] CMR provides characteristic imaging of the structural changes and tissue characterization in patients with cardiac amyloidosis with features of high native T1, expanded ECV, and diffuse subendocardial or patchy LGE Post-gadolinium myocardial signal intensity changes characteristically with myocardial signal nulling before the blood pool signal in amyloidosis and vice versa in non-amyloid hearts.[112]

Glycogen storage disease is a heterogeneous group of inherited metabolic disorders characterized by abnormalities in the enzymes that regulate the synthesis or degradation of glycogen and typically affecting males. Some of them imply heart involvement. Cardiac manifestations include severe LV hypertrophy and restrictive cardiomyopathy with HFpEF. In advanced stages, dilated cardiomyopathy occurs.[113] CMR may help in determining etiology, particularly differentiating these forms from hypertrophic cardiomyopathy.[114,115] Sarcoidosis is a multisystem granulomatous disease of unknown etiology, that can affect any organ in the body, and principally women. Although typically involving the lungs, the heart is a target in 5-7% of cases and strongly impacts survival.[116] Cardiac sarcoidosis (CS) has three successive histological stages: edema, noncaseating granulomatous infiltration, and patchy myocardial fibrosis. CMR can demonstrate early signs of myocardial infiltration in CS before more routine imaging modalities, such as scintigraphy or echocardiography and can be utilized as the first imaging modality. This is important since successful diagnosis can lead to the early initiation of steroid therapy can prevent ventricular remodeling and reduce the risk of ventricular tachyarrhythmias.[117–119] Even though various patterns of LGE can be seen, CS on CMR usually leads to patchy and multifocal LGE in noncoronary distribution. Typically, this includes subepicardial and midwall LGE rarely subendocardial pattern along the basal septum, sometimes with extension into the right ventricular insertion points as well as the inferolateral wall.[120] In patients with known or suspected CS, RV ejection fraction and RV LGE at CMR are both associated with adverse events. Furthermore, RV LGE shows good discrimination in identifying these patients at high risk of sudden cardiac death.[121]

SUMMARY

The influence of gender in HFpEF is of utmost importance as cardiac physiology, response to the immune system, hormonal balance, cardiovascular risk factors affecting myocardial structure and function are different in women compare to men. Imaging is a powerful and essential tool not only for diagnosis but also to underline the subtle sex-related differences, which could lead to better phenotype and better management of the disease. In this framework, a multi-modality approach can lead to optimal diagnostic evaluation and management of women with HFpEF.

CLINICS CARE POINTS

- Sex related differences are typical among HFpEF patients, as cardiac physiology, cardiovascular risk factors, immune system, and hormonal balance lead to different phenotypes of HFpEF.

- Imaging can play a role in underlying these gender differences.
- A multi modality imaging approach could help in performing a correct diagnosis and in observing gender differences in the severity of the disease and in the grade of diastolic dysfunction.

DISCLOSURE

The authors have nothing to disclose.

REFERENCES

1. Behnoush AH, Khalaji A, Naderi N, et al. ACC/AHA/HFSA 2022 and ESC 2021 guidelines on heart failure comparison. ESC Heart Failure 2023. https://doi.org/10.1002/ehf2.14255.

2. Gori M, Lam CSP, Gupta DK, et al. Sex-specific cardiovascular structure and function in heart failure with preserved ejection fraction. Eur J Heart Fail 2014;16:535–42.

3. Gori M, D'Elia E, Zambelli G, et al. Heart Failure with preserved ejection fraction: an update on diagnosis and treatment. G Ital Cardiol 2020;21:119–27.

4. Abramov D, Kettleson M. The universal definition of heart failure: strenght and opportunities. J Card Fail 2021;6:622–4.

5. Gori M, D'Elia E, Iorio A, et al. Clinical application of personalized medicine: heart failure with preserved left ventricular ejection fraction. Eur Heart J Suppl 2020;22:L124–8.

6. McDonagh TA, Metra M, Adamo M, et al. 2021 ESC guidelines for the diagnosis and treatment of acute and chronic heart failure. Eur Heart J 2021;42:3599–726.

7. Vadya GN, Abramov D. Echocardiografic evaluation of diastolic function is of limited value in the diagnosis and management of HFpEF. J Card Fail 2018;6:392–6.

8. Pieske B, Tschöpe C, de Boer RA, et al. How to diagnose heart failure with preserved ejection fraction: the HFA–PEFF diagnostic algorithm: a consensus recommendation from the Heart Failure Association (HFA) of the European Society of Cardiology. ESC Eur H Jour 2019;40:3297–317.

9. Abramov D, Purvi P. Diving into the diagnostic scores algorithm for Heart Failure with preserved ejection fraction. Abramov D, Parvani P. Front Cardiovasc Med 2021;8:665424.

10. Gevaert AB, Kataria R, Zannad F, et al. Heart failure with preserved ejection fraction: recent concepts in diagnosis, mechanisms and management. Heart 2022;108:1342–50.

11. Scantlebury DC, Borlaug BA. Why are women more likely than men to develop heart failure with preserved ejection fraction? Curr Opin Cardiol 2011;26:562–8.

12. Van Ommen AMLN, Canto ED, Cramer MJ, et al. Diastolic dysfunction and sex-specific progression to HFpEF: current gaps in knowledge and future directions. BMC Med 2022;20:496.

13. Wood PW, Choy JB, Nanda NC, et al. Left ventricular ejection fraction and volumes: it depends on the imaging method. Echocardiography 2014;31:87–100.

14. Owan TE, Hodge DO, Herges RM, et al. Trends in prevalence and outcome of heart failure with preserved ejection fraction. N Engl J Med 2006;355:251–9.

15. Savji N, Meijers WC, Bartz TM, et al. The association of obesity and cardiometabolic traits with incident HFpEF and HFrEF. JACC Hear Fail 2018;6:701–9.

16. Magnussen C, Niiranen TJ, Ojeda FM, et al. Sex-specific epidemiology of heart failure risk and mortality in Europe: results from the BiomarCaRE Consortium. JACC Hear Fail 2019;7:204–13.

17. Sotomi Y, Hikoso S, Nakatani D, et al. Sex differences in heart failure with preserved ejection fraction. J Am Heart Assoc 2021;10:10.

18. Beale AL, Cosentino C, Segan L, et al. The effect of parity on exercise physiology in women with heart failure with preserved ejection fraction. ESC Heart Fail 2020;7:213–22.

19. Zhao Z, Wang H, Jessup JA, et al. Role of estrogen in diastolic dysfunction. Am J Physiol Heart Circ Physiol 2014;306:H628–40.

20. Klein SL, Flanagan KL. Sex differences in immune responses. Nat Rev Immunol 2016;16:626–38.

21. Beale AL, Meyer P, Marwick TH, et al. Sex differences in cardiovascular pathophysiology: why women are overrepresented in heart failure with preserved ejection fraction. Circulation 2018;138:198–205.

22. Beale AL, Nanayakkara S, Segan L, et al. Sex differences in heart failure with preserved ejection fraction pathophysiology: a detailed invasive hemodynamic and echocardiographic analysis. JACC Heart Fail 2019;7:239–49.

23. Keskin M, Avsar S, Hayiroglu MI, et al. Relation of the number of parity to left ventricular diastolic function in pregnancy. Am J Cardiol 2017;120:154–9.

24. Leo I, Nakou E, de Marvao A, et al. Imaging in women with heart failure: sex-specific characteristics and current challenges. Card Fail Rev 2022;8:e29.

25. Vidula MK, Bravo PE, Chirinos JA. The role of multimodality imaging in the evaluation of heart failure with preserved ejection fraction. Cardiol Clin 2022;40:443–57.

26. Grilo GA, Shaver PR, Stoffel HJ, et al. Age and sex dependent differences in extracellular matrix metabolism associated with cardiac functional and structural changes. J Mol Cell Cardiol 2020;139: 62–74.

27. Gebhard C, Buechel RR, Stähli BE, et al. Impact of age and sex on left ventricular function determined by coronary computed tomographic angiography: results from the prospective multicentre CONFIRM study. Eur Heart J Cardiovasc Imaging 2017;18: 990–1000.

28. Chung AK, Das SR, Leonard D, et al. Women have higher left ventricular ejection fractions than men independent of differences in left ventricular volume: the Dallas Heart Study. Circulation 2006; 113:1597–604.

29. Redfield MM, Jacobsen SJ, Borlaug BA, et al. Age- and gender-related ventricular-vascular stiffening: a community based study. Circulation 2005;112: 2254–62.

30. Le Ven F, Bibeau K, De Larochellière É, et al. Cardiac morphology and function reference values derived from a large subset of healthy young Caucasian adults by magnetic resonance imaging. Eur Heart J Cardiovasc Imaging 2016;17:981–90.

31. Kuch B, Muscholl M, Luchner A, et al. Gender specific differences in left ventricular adaptation to obesity and hypertension. J Hum Hypertens 1998;12:685–91.

32. Lieb W, Xanthakis V, Sullivan LM, et al. Longitudinal tracking of left ventricular mass over the adult life course: clinical correlates of short- and long-term change in the Framingham offspring study. Circulation 2009;119:3085–92.

33. Dalen H, Thorstensen A, Vatten LJ, et al. Reference values and distribution of conventional echocardiographic Doppler measures and longitudinal tissue Doppler velocities in a population free from cardiovascular disease. Circ Cardiovasc Imaging 2010;3: 614–22.

34. Okura H, Takada Y, Yamabe A, et al. Age- and gender-specific changes in the left ventricular relaxation: a Doppler echocardiographic study in healthy individuals. Circ Cardiovasc Imaging 2009;2:41–6.

35. Dewan P, Rørth R, Raparelli V, et al. Sex-related differences in heart failure with preserved ejection fraction. Circ Heart Fail 2019;12:e006539.

36. Quarta G, Gori M, Iorio A, et al. Cardiac magnetic resonance in heart failure with preserved ejection fraction: myocyte,interstitium, microvascular, and metabolic abnormalities. Eur J Heart Fail 2020;22: 1065–75.

37. Bucciarelli-Ducci C, Ostenfeld E, Baldassarre LA, et al. Cardiovascular disease in women: insights from magnetic resonance imaging. J Cardiovasc Magn Reson 2020;22:71.

38. Petersen SE, Aung N, Sanghvi MM, et al. Reference ranges for cardiac structure and function using cardiovascular magnetic resonance (CMR) in Caucasians from the UK biobank population cohort. J Cardiovasc Magn Reson 2017; 19:18.

39. Maceira AM, Prasad SK, Khan M, et al. Normalized left ventricular systolic and diastolic function by steady state free precession cardiovascular magnetic resonance. J Cardiovasc Magn Reson 2006; 8:417–26.

40. Alfakih K, Plein S, Thiele H, et al. Normal human left and right ventricular dimensions for MRI as assessed by turbo gradient echo and steady-state free precession imaging sequences. J Magn Reson Imaging 2003;17:323–9.

41. Petersen SE, Khanji MY, Plein S, et al. European Association of Cardiovascular Imaging expert consensus paper: a comprehensive review of cardiovascular magnetic resonance normal values of cardiac chamber size and aortic root in adults and recommendations for grading severity. Eur Heart J Cardiovasc Imaging 2019;20:1321–31.

42. Franssen C, Miqueo AG. The role of titin and extracellular matrix remodeling in heart failure with preserved ejection fraction. Neth Heart J 2016;24: 259–67.

43. Obokata M, Olson TP, Reddy YNV, et al. Hemodynamics, dyspnea, and pulmonary reserve in heart failure with preserved ejection fraction. Eur Heart J 2018;39:2810.

44. Kawel-Bohem N, Hetzel SJ, Ambale-Venkatesh B, et al. Reference ranges ("normal values") for cardiovascular magnetic resonance (CMR) in adults and children: 2020 update. Jour Cardiac Magn Res 2020;22:87.

45. Haaf P, Garg P, Messroghli D, et al. Cardiac T1 mapping and extracellular volume (ECV) in clinical practice: a comprehensive review. J Cardiovasc Magn Reson 2016;18:89.

46. Nelson M. Left ventricular diastolic dysfunction in women with nonobstructive ischemic heart disease: insights from magnetic resonance imaging and spectroscopy. Am J Physiol Regul Integr Comp Physiol 2017;313:R322–9.

47. Schelbert EB, Miller CA. Myocardial tissue characteristics undoubtedly differ by gender but not age. European Heart Journal - Cardiovascular Imaging 2018;19:611–2.

48. Blaaha MJ, DeFilippis AP. Multi-ethnic study of atherosclerosis (MESA). J Am Coll Cardiol 2021; 77:3195–216.

49. Reis SE, Holubkov R, Smith A, et al. Coronary microvascular dysfunction is highly prevalent in women with chest pain in the absence of coronary artery disease: results from the NHLBI WISE study. Am Heart J 2001;141:735–41.

50. Pepine CJ, Petersen JW, Merz CNB. A microvascular-myocardial diastolic dysfunctional state and risk for mental stress ischemia: a revised concept of ischemia during daily life. JACC (J Am Coll Cardiol): Cardiovascular Imaging 2014;7: 362–5.

51. Paulus WJ, Tschöpe C. A novel paradigm for heart failure with preserved ejection fraction: co-morbidities drive myocardial dysfunction and re-modeling through coronary microvascular endothelial inflammation. J Am Coll Cardiol 2013;62:263–71.

52. Pathik B, Raman B, Mohd Amin NH, et al. Troponin-positive chest pain with unobstructed coronary arteries: incremental diagnostic value of cardiovascular magnetic resonance imaging. Eur Heart J Cardiovasc Imaging 2016;17:1146–52.

53. Bakir M, Wei J, Nelson MD, et al. Cardiac magnetic resonance imaging for myocardial perfusion and diastolic function—reference control values for women. Cardiovasc Diagn Ther 2016;6:78–86.

54. Mauricio R, Srichai MB, Axel L, et al. Stress cardiac MRI in women with myocardial infarction and non-obstructive coronary artery disease. Clin Cardiol 2016;39:596–602.

55. Dastidar AG, Baritussio A, De Garate E, et al. Prognostic role of cardiac MRI and conventional risk factors in myocardial infarction with non-obstructed coronary arteries. J Am Coll Cardiol Img 2019;12:1973–82.

56. Gorcsan J 3rd, Tanaka H. Echocardiographic assessment of myocardial strain. J Am Coll Cardiol 2011;58:1401–13.

57. Petersen JW, Nazir TF, Lee L, et al. Speckle tracking echocardiography-determined measures of global and regional left ventricular function correlate with functional capacity in patients with and without preserved ejection fraction. Cardiovasc Ultrasound 2013;11:20.

58. Kraigher-Krainer E, Shah AM, Gupta DK, et al. Investigators P. Impaired systolic function by strain imaging in heart failure with preserved ejection fraction. J Am Coll Cardiol 2014;63: 447–56.

59. Pellicori P, Kallvikbacka-Bennett A, Khaleva O, et al. Global longitudinal strain in patients with suspected heart failure and a normal ejection fraction: does it improve diagnosis and risk stratification? Int J Cardiovasc Imag 2014;30:69–79.

60. Buggey J, Alenezi F, Yoon HY, et al. Left ventricular global longitudinal strain in patients with heart failure with preserved ejection fraction: outcomes following an acute heart failure hospitalization. ESC Heart Failure 2017;4:432–9.

61. Cao Y, Vergnes L, Wang YC, et al. Sex differences in heart mitochondria regulate diastolic dysfunction. Nat Commun 2022;13:3850.

62. Yoneyama A, Koyama J, Tomita T, et al. Relationship of plasma brain-type natriuretic peptide levels to left ventricular longitudinal function in patients with congestive heart failure assessed by strain Doppler imaging. Int J Cardiol 2008;130:56–63.

63. Shah AM, Claggett B, Sweitzer NK, et al. The prognostic importance of impaired systolic function in heart failure with preserved ejection fraction and the impact of spironolactone. Circulation 2015; 132:402–14.

64. Wang J, Fang F, Wai-Kwok Yip G, et al. Left ventricular long axis performance during exercise is an important prognosticator in patients with heart failure and preserved ejection fraction. Int J Cardiol 2014;178C:131–5.

65. Stampehl MR, Mann DL, Nguyen JS, et al. Speckle strain echocardiography predicts outcome in patients with heart failure with both depressed and preserved left ventricular ejection fraction. Echocardiography 2015;32:71–8.

66. Reddy YNV, Obokata M, Egbe A, et al. Left atrial strain and compliance in the diagnostic evaluation of heart failure with preserved ejection fraction. Eur J Heart Fail 2019;21:891–900.

67. Von Roeder M, Rommel KP, Kowallick JT, et al. Influence of left atrial function on exercise capacity and left ventricular function in patients with heart failure and preserved ejection fraction. Circ Cardiovasc Imaging 2017;10:e005467.

68. Zhang S, Shou Y, Han S, et al. The diagnostic and prognostic value of cardiac magnetic resonance strain analysis in heart failure with preserved ejection fraction. Contrast Media Mol Imaging 2023;8: 5996741.

69. Kurt M, Wang J, Torre-Amione G, et al. Left atrial function in diastolic heart failure. Circ Cardiovasc Imaging 2009;2:10–5.

70. Obokata M, Negishi K, Kurosawa K, et al. Incremental diagnostic value of la strain with leg lifts in heart failure with preserved ejection fraction. JACC Cardiovasc Imaging 2013;6:749–58.

71. Khan MS, Memon MM, Murad MH, et al. Left atrial function in heart failure with preserved ejection fraction: a systematic review and meta-analysis. Eur J Heart Fail 2020;22:472–85.

72. Sanchis L, Gabrielli L, Andrea R, et al. Left atrial dysfunction relates to symptom onset in patients with heart failure and preserved left ventricular ejection fraction. Eur Heart Cardiovasc Imaging 2015;16:62–7.

73. Sanchis L, La Garza MS, Bijnens B, et al. Gender influence on the adaptation of atrial performance to training. Eur J Sport Sci 2017;17:720–6.

74. Truong VT, Palmer C, Wolking S, et al. Normal left atrial strain and strain rate using cardiac magnetic resonance feature tracking in healthy volunteers. Eur Heart J Cardiovasc Imaging 2020;21:446–53.

75. Qu YY, Buckert D, Ma GS, et al. Quantitative assessment of left and right atrial strains using cardiovascular magnetic resonance based tissue tracking. Front Cardiovasc Med 2021;8:690240.

76. Eckstein J, Körperich H, Paluszkiewicz L, et al. Multi-parametric analyses to investigate dependencies of normal left atrial strain by cardiovascular magnetic resonance feature tracking. Sci Rep 2022;12:12233.

77. Koutsampasopoulos K, Vogiatzis I, Ziakas A, et al. Right ventricular performance in patients with heart failure with mildly reduced ejection fraction: the forgotten ventricle. Int J Cardiovasc Imag 2022; 38:2363–72.

78. Galiè N, Humbert M, Vachiery JL, et al. 2015 ESC/ERS guidelines for the diagnosis and treatment of pulmonary hypertension: The joint task force for the diagnosis and treatment of pulmonary hypertension of the European society of cardiology (ESC) and the European respiratory society (ERS): Endorsed by: Association for European paediatric and congenital cardiology (AEPC), international society for heart and lung transplantation (ISHLT). Eur Heart J 2016;37:67–119.

79. Rudski LG, Lai WW, Afilalo J, et al. Guidelines for the echocardiographic assessment of the right heart in adults: a report from the American Society of Echocardiography endorsed by the European Association of Echocardiography, a registered branch of the European Society of Cardiology, and the Canadian Society of Echocardiography. J Am Soc Echocardiogr 2010;23:685–713 [quiz: 786-788].

80. Howard LS, Grapsa J, Dawson D, et al. Echocardiographic assessment of pulmonary hypertension: standard operating procedure. Eur Respir Rev 2012;21:239–48.

81. Greiner S, Jud A, Aurich M, et al. Reliability of noninvasive assessment of systolic pulmonary artery pressure by Doppler echocardiography compared to right heart catheterization: analysis in a large patient population. J Am Heart Assoc 2014;3:e001103.

82. Hur DJ, Sugeng L. Non-invasive multimodality cardiovascular imaging of the right heart and pulmonary circulation in pulmonary hypertension. Front Cardiovasc Med 2019;6:24.

83. Dalto M, Romeo E, Argiento P. Pulmonary arterial hypertension: the key role of echocardiography. Echocardiography 2015;32(Suppl 1):S23–37.

84. Singh I, Oliveira RKF, Heerdt PM, et al. Sex-related differences in dynamic right ventricular-pulmonary vascular coupling in heart failure with preserved ejection fraction. Chest 2021;159:2402–16.

85. Nitsche C, Kammerlander AA, Binder C, et al. Mascherbauer J Native T1 time of right ventricular insertion points by cardiac magnetic resonance: relation with invasive haemodynamics and outcome in heart failure with preserved ejection fraction. Eur Heart J Cardiovasc Imaging 2020;2: 683–769.

86. Aschauer S, Kammerlander AA, Zotter-Tufaro C, et al. The right heart in heart failure with preserved ejection fraction: insights from cardiac magnetic resonance imaging and invasive haemodynamics: The right heart in heart failure with preserved ejection fraction. Eur J Heart Fail 2016;18:71–80.

87. Humbert M, Kovacs G, Hoeper MM, et al. 2022 ESC/ERS Guidelines for the diagnosis and treatment of pulmonary hypertension. Eur Heart J 2022;43:3618–731.

88. Hachulla E, Gressin V, Guillevin L, et al. Early detection of pulmonary arterial hypertension in systemic sclerosis: a French nationwide prospective multicenter study. Arthritis Rheum 2005;52:3792–800.

89. Kawut SM, Lima JAC, Barr RG, et al. Sex and race differences in right ventricular structure and function: the MESA-right ventricle study. Circulation 2011;123:2542–51.

90. Ostenfeld E, Stephensen SS, Steding-Ehrenborg K, et al. Regional contribution to ventricular stroke volume is affected on the left side, but not on the right in patients with pulmonary hypertension. Int J Cardiovasc Imag 2016;32:1243–53.

91. van Wolferen SA, Marcus JT, Boonstra A, et al. Prognostic value of right ventricular mass, volume, and function in idiopathic pulmonary arterial hypertension. Eur Heart J 2007;28:1250–7.

92. Freed BH, Gomberg-Maitland M, Chandra S, et al. Late gadolinium enhancement cardiovascular magnetic resonance predicts clinical worsening in patients with pulmonary hypertension. J Cardiovasc Magn Reson 2012;14:11.

93. Sanz J, Dellegrottaglie S, Kariisa M, et al. Prevalence and correlates of septal delayed contrast enhancement in patients with pulmonary hypertension. Am J Cardiol 2007;100:731–5.

94. Blyth KG, Groenning BA, Martin TN, et al. Contrast enhanced-cardiovascular magnetic resonance imaging in patients with pulmonary hypertension. Eur Heart J 2005;26:1993–9.

95. Jacobs W, van de Veerdonk MC, Trip P, et al. The right ventricle explains sex differences in survival in idiopathic pulmonary arterial hypertension. Chest 2014;145:1230–6.

96. Chin KM, Kingman M, de Lemos JA, et al. Changes in right ventricular structure and function assessed using cardiac magnetic resonance imaging in bosentan-treated patients with pulmonary arterial hypertension. Am J Cardiol 2008;101:1669–72.

97. Lau ES, Cunningham T, Hardin KM, et al. Sex differences in cardiometabolic traits and determinants of exercise capacity in heart failure with preserved ejection fraction. JAMA Cardiol 2020;5:30–7.

98. Petre RE, Quaile MP, Rossman EI, et al. Sex-based differences in myocardial contractile reserve. Am J Physiol Regul Integr Comp Physiol 2007;292: R810–8.

99. Pugliese NR, De Biase N, Del Punta L, et al. Deep phenotype characterization of hypertensive response to exercise: implications on functional capacity and prognosis across the heart failure spectrum. Eur J Heart Fail 2023;25:497–509.

100. Omar AMS, Konje S, Munoz Estrella A, et al. Prognostic significance of incorporating exercise tissue doppler mitral annular early diastolic velocity in exercise diastolic dysfunction assessment. Echocardiography 2023;40:397–407.

101. Malhotra R, Bakken K, D'Elia E, et al. Cardiopulmonary exercise testing in heart failure. JAC Heart Fail 2016;4:607–17.

102. Rozenbaum Z, Granot Y, Sadeh B, et al. Sex differences in heart failure patients assessed by combined echocardiographic and cardiopulmonary exercise testing. Front Cardiovasc Med 2023;10: 1098395.

103. Jung MH, Ihm SH, Lee DH, et al. Sex-specific associations of obesity with exercise capacity and diastolic function in Koreans. Nutr Metab Cardiovasc Dis 2021;31:254–62.

104. Honigberg MC, Lau ES, Jones AD, et al. Sex differences in exercise capacity and quality of life in heart failure with preserved ejection fraction: a secondary analysis of the RELAX and NEAT-HFpEF trials. J Card Fail 2020;26:276–80.

105. Lee E, Ibrahim EH, Parwani P, et al. Practical guide to evaluating myocardial disease by cardiac MRI. AJR Am J Roentgenol 2020;214:546–56.

106. Sipe JD, Benson MD, Buxbaum JN, et al. Amyloid fibril proteins and amyloidosis: chemical identification and clinical classification. International Society of Amyloidosis 2016 Nomenclature Guidelines. Amyloid 2016;23:209–13.

107. Merlini G, Palladini G. Light chain amyloidosis: the heart of the problem. Haematologica 2013;98: 1492–5.

108. Ruberg FL, Berk JL. Transthyretin (TTR) cardiac amyloidosis. Circulation 2012;126:1286–300.

109. Jaiswal V, Ang SP, Chia JE, et al. Echocardiographic predictors of presence of cardiac amyloidosis in aortic stenosis. Eur Heart J Cardiovasc Imaging 2022;23:1290–301.

110. Agha AM, Parwani P, Guha A, et al. Role of cardiovascular imaging for the diagnosis and prognosis of cardiac amyloidosis. Open Heart 2018;5(2): e000881.

111. Dorbala S, Cuddy S, Falk RH. How to image cardiac amyloidosis: a practical approach. JACC Cardiovasc Imaging 2020;13:1368–83.

112. Mousavi N, Cheezum MK, Aghayev A, et al. Assessment of cardiac masses by cardiac magnetic resonance imaging: histological correlation and clinical outcomes. J Am Heart Assoc 2019;8: e007829.

113. O'Hanlon R, Pennell DJ. Cardiovascular magnetic resonance in the evaluation of hypertrophic and infiltrative cardiomyopathies. Heart Fail Clin 2009; 5:369–87.

114. Moon JC, Mundy HR, Lee PJ, et al. Myocardial fibrosis in glycogen storage disease type III. Circulation 2003;107:e47.

115. Arad M, Maron BJ, Gorham JM, et al. Glycogen storage diseases presenting as hypertrophic cardiomyopathy. N Engl J Med 2005;352:362–72.

116. Roberts W, McAllister H, Ferrans V. Sarcoidosis of the heart: a clinicopathologic study of 35 necropsy patients (group 1) and review of 78 previously described necropsy patients (group II). Am J Med 1977;63:86–108.

117. Bargout R, Kelly RF. Sarcoid heart disease: clinical course and treatment. Int J Cardiol 2004;97: 173–82.

118. Vignaux O, Dhote R, Duboc D, et al. Clinical significance of myocardial magnetic resonance abnormalities in patients with sarcoidosis: a 1-year follow-up study. Chest 2002;122:1895–901.

119. Rosenthal DG, Parwani P, Murray TO, et al. Long-term corticosteroid-sparing immunosuppression for cardiac sarcoidosis. J Am Heart Assoc 2019; 8(18).

120. Parwani P, Patel AR. Diagnostic testing in cardiac sarcoidosis: what comes first? J Nucl Cardiol 2023. https://doi.org/10.1007/s12350-023-03257-9.

121. Wang J, Zhang J, Hosadurg N, et al. Prognostic value of RV abnormalities on CMR in patients with known or suspected cardiac sarcoidosis. JACC Cardiovasc Imaging 2023;16:361–72.

Evaluation and Management of Cardiac Sarcoidosis with Advanced Imaging

Rishi Shrivastav, MD[a], Adrija Hajra, MD, MRCP[b], Suraj Krishnan, MD[c,1],
Dhrubajyoti Bandyopadhyay, MD[d], Pragya Ranjan, MD[d,*],
Anthon Fuisz, MD[d]

KEYWORDS

- Cardiac sarcoidosis • Echocardiography
- Single-photon emission computerized tomography (SPECT)
- Cardiac magnetic resonance imaging (MRI) • 18F-FDG PET • Late gadolinium enhancement (LGE)

KEY POINTS

- Cardiac imaging is an indispensable tool in diagnosing and managing cardiac sarcoidosis when used in the appropriate clinical setting.
- Echocardiography is relatively cheap, easily available, and rapidly performed imaging modality when clinical suspicion is high. Abnormal findings, however, are neither sensitive nor specific.
- Cardiac magnetic resonance imaging (MRI) is often the first screening test employed with advanced imaging. The most common findings include the presence of late gadolinium enhancement (LGE) in the mid-myocardial pattern, which also has a prognostic value.
- ^{18}F-Fluorodeoxyglucose (^{18}F-FDG) positron emission tomography (PET) performed in combination with myocardial perfusion imaging often detects the presence of active inflammation and helps in the staging of disease and response to therapy.
- When cardiac MRI and ^{18}F-FDG PET are combined, the sensitivity and specificity to diagnose cardiac sarcoidosis are the highest.

INTRODUCTION

Sarcoidosis is a systemic granulomatous disease of unknown etiology with heterogeneous clinical manifestations. It mainly affects adults in the third and fourth decade of life with a second peak, especially in women over 50 with variable clinical presentation influenced by geographic, ethnic, and environmental factors.[1,2] Its first modern description is attributed to James Hutchinson in 1869.[3,4] In most cases, it affects the lungs and intrathoracic lymph nodes. However, other organs, including the skin, eyes, liver, heart, and nervous system are affected with variable clinical presentations.[5] The pathophysiology of sarcoidosis is not clear. The clinical manifestations are

[a] Department of Cardiology, Icahn School of Medicine at Mount Sinai/Mount Sinai Morningside Hospital, Cardiovascular Institute, 1111 Amsterdam Avenue, Clark Building, 2nd Floor, New York, NY 10023, USA;
[b] Department of Internal Medicine, Montefiore Medical Center/Albert Einstein College of Medicine, 1825 Eastchester Road, Bronx, NY 10461, USA; [c] Department of Internal Medicine, Jacobi Hospital/Albert Einstein College of Medicine, Bronx, NY, USA; [d] Department of Cardiology, New York Medical College, Westchester Medical Center, 100 Woods Road, Valhalla, NY 10595, USA
[1] Present address: 1680 Pelham Parkway South, Apartment 112, Bronx, NY 10461.
* Corresponding author.
E-mail address: pragya.503@gmail.com

Heart Failure Clin 19 (2023) 475–489
https://doi.org/10.1016/j.hfc.2023.06.002

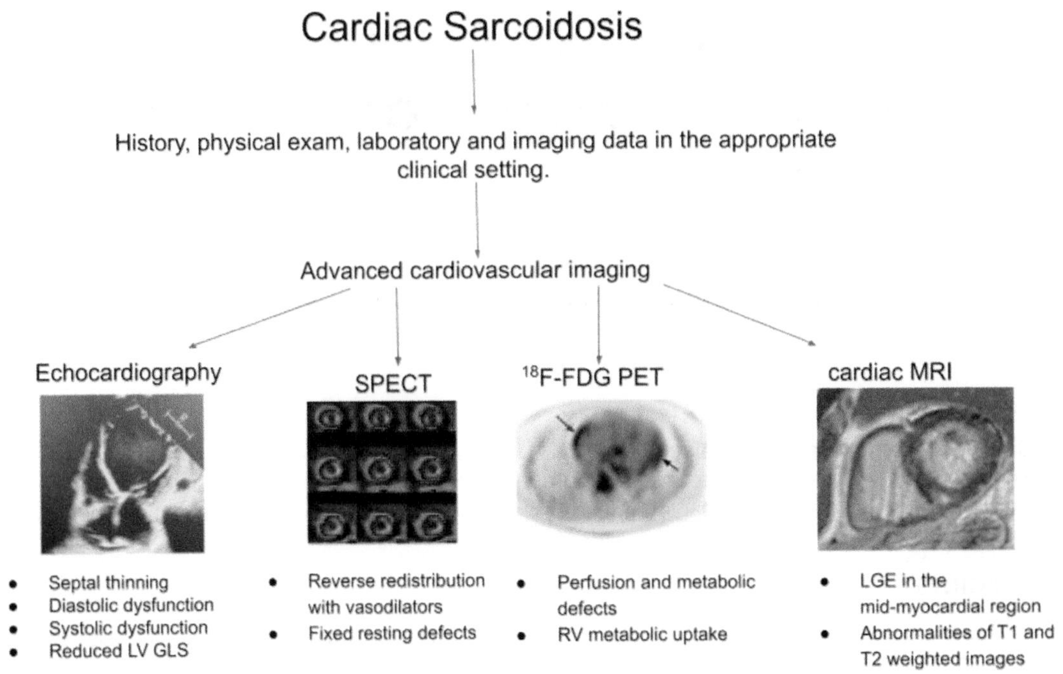

Cardiac Sarcoidosis

History, physical exam, laboratory and imaging data in the appropriate clinical setting.

Advanced cardiovascular imaging

| Echocardiography | SPECT | 18F-FDG PET | cardiac MRI |

- Septal thinning
- Diastolic dysfunction
- Systolic dysfunction
- Reduced LV GLS

- Reverse redistribution with vasodilators
- Fixed resting defects

- Perfusion and metabolic defects
- RV metabolic uptake

- LGE in the mid-myocardial region
- Abnormalities of T1 and T2 weighted images

Fig. 1. Central Illustration. 18F FDG-PET, positron emission tomography with 2-deoxy-2-[fluorine-18] fluoro-D-glucose; LGE, late gadolinium enhancement; LV GLS, left ventricular global longitudinal strain; MRI, magnetic resonance imaging; RV, right ventricle; SPECT, single-photon emission computerized tomography. The (arrows) show the different options for advanced imaging.

mostly non-specific. Given the multi-organ involvement, patients with sarcoidosis can present with various presentations. The pulmonary system is most involved, but cardiac manifestations are also noted in patients with sarcoidosis.[5] Cardiac involvement is often underdiagnosed. Missed diagnosis at the early stage of cardiac sarcoidosis (CS) can put patients at risk of developing cardiac complications, including heart block, arrhythmias, heart failure (HF), and sudden cardiac death. The lack of specific symptoms and signs and poor sensitivity of tissue biopsy makes imaging modalities an essential diagnostic tool for CS.[6] In this article, the authors have discussed the epidemiology and pathophysiology of CS, emphasizing different imaging modalities, particularly advanced imaging techniques, used for early diagnosis, staging, prognosis, follow-up, and determination of complications of CS.

EPIDEMIOLOGY

Sarcoidosis is prevalent worldwide, with the highest prevalence in the Nordic, African- American and economically disadvantaged populations.[7,8] The disease is more common in females than males, with a higher predilection in non-smokers than smokers.[8] In many cases, CS remains subclinical until the late stages of the disease.[9]

Clinically, CS has been noted in 5% of patients with systemic sarcoidosis. In comparison, autopsy studies have found cardiac involvement in up to 25% of Caucasian and African American patients and up to 80% of Japanese patients.[9–11] Epidemiologic data suggest cardiac involvement of sarcoidosis may be more commonly seen in men than women, who manifest symptoms and signs of systemic sarcoidosis more often.[9,12] Moreover, sarcoidosis rarely occurs with isolated cardiac involvement without affecting other organ systems.[13,14]

CLINICAL PRESENTATION AND COMPLICATIONS OF CARDIAC SARCOIDOSIS

Patients with sarcoidosis can present with non-specific complaints of systemic inflammation such as fever, malaise, night sweats, and weight loss.[15,16] Since any part of the heart can be affected in CS, the clinical symptoms will vary based on disease focus and extent. Involvement of interventricular septum and LV commonly result in conduction abnormalities, cardiomyopathy, or tachyarrhythmias presenting as fatigue, syncope, palpitations, or sudden cardiac death.[17] Sudden cardiac death can occur secondary to progressive conduction abnormalities and ventricular arrhythmias in 25% to 65% of cases and could be isolated presentations in 14% of cases.[5,18] Inflammation and fibrosis from CS can compromise heart function, causing HF symptoms in less than 20% of cases.[19–21] RV involvement can occur alongside LV involvement though isolated RV involvement is rare. CS involving RV can increase the risk of arrhythmia and RV systolic dysfunction, which itself portends a poor prognosis.[5,22]

EXISTING CRITERIA FOR THE DIAGNOSIS OF CARDIAC SARCOIDOSIS

CS is diagnosed with a combination of clinical, histologic, and imaging modalities. The two main diagnostic criteria used for CS are the Heart Rhythm Society (HRS) 2014 guidelines and the Japanese Circulation Society (JCS) 2016 guidelines, summarized in **Table 1**. One of the major differences between the two guidelines is the inclusion of diagnostic criteria for isolated CS in JCS 2016 guidelines. The diagnosis of isolated CS can be made when no clinical characteristics

of sarcoidosis are observed in any organs other than the heart along with an absence of imaging evidence of other organ involvement on chest CT, Gallium-67 (Ga-67) scintigraphy or positron emission tomography with 2-deoxy-2-[fluorine-18] fluoro- D-glucose (18F-FDG PET). The evolution of diagnostic criteria for CS shows the growing reliance on advanced cardiac imaging in diagnosing CS. Of note, the patchy involvement of the layers of the heart, typically the sub-epicardium or the mid-wall distribution of CS lesions, markedly decreases the sensitivity of blind endomyocardial biopsy for CS. Imaging-guided procedures or electro-anatomical mapping may increase sensitivity, though further validation of these approaches is needed.[15,16]

IMAGING APPROACH TO CARDIAC SARCOIDOSIS

The diagnosis of CS is always challenging given the absence of specific and typical symptoms,

---

Table 1
Diagnostic guidelines for cardiac sarcoidosis

HRS 2014 Expert Consensus	JCS 2016 Guidelines
1. Histologic Diagnosis from Myocardial Tissue	1. Histologic diagnosis group
CS is diagnosed in the presence of non-caseating granuloma on histologic examination of myocardial tissue with no alternative cause identified (including negative organismal stains if applicable).	CS is diagnosed histologically when endomyocardial biopsy or surgical specimens demonstrate non-caseating epithelioid granulomas and when granulomas due to other causes and local sarcoid reactions can be ruled out.
2. Clinical Diagnosis from Invasive and Non-Invasive Studies	2. Clinical diagnosis group (negative myocardial biopsy findings or those not undergoing myocardial biopsy)
a. There is a histologic diagnosis of extra-cardiac sarcoidosis and b. One or more of the following is present • Steroid ± immunosuppressant responsive cardiomyopathy or heart block • Unexplained reduced LVEF (40%) • Unexplained sustained (spontaneous or induced) VT • Mobitz type II 2nd degree heart block or 3rd degree heart block • Patchy uptake on dedicated cardiac PET (in a pattern consistent with CS) • Late Gadolinium Enhancement on CMR (in a pattern consistent with CS) • Positive gallium uptake (in a pattern consistent with CS)	1. When epithelioid granulomas are found in organs other than the heart, and clinical findings strongly suggestive of cardiac involvement are present*. 2. When the patient shows clinical findings strongly suggestive of pulmonary or ophthalmic sarcoidosis & at least 2 of the five characteristic laboratory findings of sarcoidosis: - • Bilateral hilar lymphadenopathy • High serum angiotensin-converting enzyme (ACE) activity or elevated serum lysozyme levels -High serum soluble interleukin-2 receptor (sIL-2R) levels • Significant tracer accumulation in 67 Gallium citrate scintigraphy or 18F-FDG PET • A high percentage of lymphocytes with a CD4/CD8 ratio of >3.5 in BAL fluid.

Abbreviations: 18F FDG-PET, Positron emission tomography with 2-deoxy-2-[fluorine-18] fluoro- D-glucose; CMR, cardiac magnetic resonance imaging; HRS, heart rhythm society; JCS, Japanese circulation society; LVEF, left ventricular ejection fraction; PET, positron emission tomography; VT, ventricular tachycardia.
   Data from Refs.[15,16]

lack of validated diagnostic tests, and low yield of endomyocardial biopsy.[23] Hence, imaging as one of the diagnostic modalities plays an important role. Four out of the five major criteria established by the Japanese Society of Sarcoidosis and other Granulomatous Disorders (JSSOG) 2015 for diagnosing CS utilized imaging to establish the diagnosis. Basal thinning of the interventricular septum or morphologic abnormality, depressed ejection fraction (EF) (<50%) or regional wall motion abnormality, abnormal uptake of Ga-67 or 18F-FDG in the heart, and late gadolinium enhancement (LGE) on cardiac magnetic resonance imaging (cMRI) are some of the important imaging findings from different modalities that aid in the diagnosis of CS.[24]

Cardiac imaging is an indispensable tool right from the early stages of disease when establishing the initial diagnosis up to the follow-up period when assessing the evolution of pathologic processes. In addition, it can help identify several complications during the disease progression and plays a vital role in gauging response to various treatments employed for managing CS.[25] Among different clinical presentations, the presence of HF strongly indicates the need for advanced therapies, including cardiac transplantation. Imaging modalities can help identify this and several other complications and add prognostic value to the overall presentation while simultaneously facilitating crucial decisions regarding patient care.[26]

Goals of Imaging

We can summarize the goal of using advanced cardiac imaging in CS as follows[27–29].

- Diagnosis of cardiac dysfunction that can be suggestive of CS.
- Diagnosis of complications associated with CS.
- Determining the prognosis of the disease, based largely on the stage and the extent of the cardiac involvement at the time of diagnosis.
- Assessment of the progression of the disease
- Assessment of the response to therapeutic regimens
- Evaluation of relapse of the disease

Diagnosis

As mentioned above, imaging findings form a crucial component of the major diagnostic criteria. **Table 1** depict the clinical, laboratory, histologic, and imaging diagnostic criteria used by HRS and the JCS in diagnosing CS.[15,16] **Table 2** describes the imaging findings to diagnose CS using JCS and HRS criteria; **Table 3** compares the salient imaging features used by these criteria.[30] We delineate the role of individual imaging modalities in the diagnosis and management of CS later in discussion.

ROLE OF ECHOCARDIOGRAPHY

Transthoracic echocardiography (TTE) is the only imaging modality recommended by HRS guidelines

Table 2
Findings on imaging used in diagnosing cardiac sarcoidosis in JCS and HRS criteria

Imaging Modality	Criteria	Findings
Echocardiography	JCS Major Criteria	Basal thinning of the interventricular septum or abnormal ventricular wall anatomy (ventricular aneurysm, thinning of the middle or upper ventricular septum, regional ventricular wall thickening) Left ventricular contractile dysfunction with LVEF<50% or focal ventricular wall asynergy
	HRS clinical diagnosis	Unexplained reduced LVEF (<40%)
18F-FDG PET	JCS Major Criteria	With abnormally high tracer accumulation in the heart
	HRS clinical diagnosis	Patchy uptake in a pattern consistent with CS
Nuclear medicine study	JCS Minor Criteria	Perfusion defects
Gadolinium-enhanced cMRI	JCS Major Criteria	Delayed contrast enhancement of the myocardium
	HRS clinical diagnosis	LGE in a pattern consistent with CS

Abbreviations: 18F-FDG-PET, positron emission tomography with 2-deoxy-2-[fluorine-18] fluoro-ᴅ-glucose; cMRI, cardiac magnetic resonance imaging; CS, cardiac sarcoidosis; HRS, Heart Rhythm Society; JCS, Japanese Circulation Society; LGE, late gadolinium enhancement; LVEF, left ventricular ejection fraction.

Adapted from Rosario KF, Brezitski K, Arps K, Milne M, Doss J, Karra R. Cardiac Sarcoidosis: Current Approaches to Diagnosis and Management. Curr Allergy Asthma Rep. 2022;22(12):171-182.

Table 3
Interpretation of the common findings on MPI and ^{18}F-FDG PET imaging

Interpretation	Perfusion Imaging	^{18}F-FDG PET Uptake
Normal	Normal	No uptake
Early disease	Normal or mild defect	Uptake in the focal area or area of defect
Mismatch pattern	Moderate to severe defect	Uptake in the area of defect
Scar Pattern	Severe defect	No or minimal uptake

Abbreviation: ^{18}F-FDG-PET, positron emission tomography with 2-deoxy-2-[fluorine-18] fluoro- D-glucose.
Data from Refs.[30,48]

to screen patients with sarcoidosis to look for cardiac involvement.[31] Although echocardiography does not have any specific finding for CS, this modality is typically the first imaging test ordered for patients clinically suspected to have possible CS.[27] TTE can be useful sometimes for diagnosing cardiac dysfunction at an early stage, even among asymptomatic patients with sarcoidosis. A cross-sectional study involving 44 asymptomatic patients with sarcoidosis showed that 3D-echocardiography-derived left atrial (LA) minimum volume indices were significantly higher in patients with sarcoidosis. The LA active EF and LA total EFs were significantly lower in the sarcoidosis group than in the control group.[32] In another study by Fahy and colleagues, up to 14% of patients with pulmonary sarcoidosis without known cardiac involvement had evidence of diastolic dysfunction attributed to CS.[33]

Two-dimensional–speckle tracking echocardiography (2D–STE) is emerging as a sensitive method for the early diagnosis of cardiac dysfunction in patients with CS. A study by Stefano and colleagues involved 83 patients with extracardiac, biopsy-proven sarcoidosis. A total of 23 patients with early-stage CS with normal LVEF and RV systolic function were found to have significantly reduced left and right ventricular global longitudinal strain (LV GLS, RV GLS) when compared with controls. LV GLS (vs control) was $-15.9\% \pm 2.5\%$ versus $-18.2\% \pm 2.7\%$; and RV GLS (vs control) was $-16.9\% \pm 4.5\%$ versus $-24.1\% \pm 4.0\%$. In the same cohort, reduced LV GLS predicted hospital admission and HF, with patients with normal strain values showing minimal adverse outcomes.[34]

The systolic dyssynchrony index (SDI) measured by three-dimensional echocardiography for 16 segments of the LV has been noted to be higher in patients with sarcoidosis compared to healthy controls in the study by Cabuk and colleagues.[35] Emerging data suggests that STE has the potential to become more sensitive than traditional echocardiography alone as a screening tool to identify patients with sarcoidosis at increased risk for cardiac involvement.[36,37]

The role of echocardiography in assessing response to treatment and therapy is limited to visualizing improvement in HF parameters such as systolic and diastolic function and strain values. Abnormalities of these parameters are independently associated with adverse short-term and long-term outcomes.[31]

ROLE OF CARDIAC SINGLE-PHOTON EMISSION COMPUTERIZED TOMOGRAPHY

Myocardial perfusion imaging (MPI) using 201 TL and 99mTc isotopes-based single-photon emission computerized tomography (SPECT) can identify focal perfusion defects at rest, which may be an indicator for the presence of cardiac sarcoidosis.[38,39] While this finding can be seen with other conditions, such as coronary artery disease and other forms of cardiomyopathy, defects attributed to CS remain fixed or demonstrate a pattern of reverse redistribution with the injection of vasodilators. A careful history and a thorough review of other tests, such as a 12-lead electrocardiogram (EKG) and coronary angiography, can help exclude some of these non-sarcoid differentials. Reverse redistribution that refers to the relative decrease in the size or, in some instances, the complete disappearance of the resting defects with stress testing or after injections of vasodilators such as dipyridamole, is observed in CS.[40] In contrast, patients with coronary ischemia demonstrate worsening of the resting defect with stress testing or injection of vasodilators. The phenomenon of reverse redistribution in CS is explained by resting microvascular vasoconstriction of the cardiac arterioles that supply part of the myocardium affected by the sarcoid granulomas, which dilate in response to vasodilator and show improved perfusion. While reverse redistribution may help differentiate CS from other forms of cardiac pathologies, such as CAD, its presence is not unique to CS alone, and caution must be used in interpretation.[41]

Adding Ga-67 scintigraphy to Thallium-201 (201 TL) and Technetium-99 (99mTc) -based cardiac SPECT may help identify regions of myocardium affected by active inflammation, assisting in recognizing the stage of the disease process. The absence of Ga-67 uptake in the region of perfusion defect may indicate a lack of active inflammation and a poor response to corticosteroid treatment.[42] However, differentiating the uptake of Ga-67 in myocardium from other body parts can often be difficult, making the application of this method challenging, not to mention the additive radiation exposure that comes with using dual isotopes.

123I-beta-methyl-p-iodophenylpentadecanoic acid (123I-BMIPP) is a 123I-based isotope taken up by healthy myocardium that utilizes free fatty acids for metabolism.[43] In sarcoid myocardium, as active inflammation and granuloma formation occur, gradual changes in myocardial metabolism shift the metabolism from free fatty acids to glucose. These changes in metabolism can be visualized as reduced 123I-BMIPP uptake within the myocardial segments affected by sarcoidosis.[44] In some instances, a reduction in 123I-BMIPP uptake may precede perfusion abnormalities, aiding in identifying the early stages of CS. Alternatively, the late stages of CS, characterized by myocardial fibrosis, are evident with defects in both perfusion and free fatty acid metabolism. Therefore, combining MPI (SPECT or PET) with 123I-BMIPP can help increase the diagnostic yield. However, since ischemic cardiomyopathy shares the same metabolic alteration as sarcoidosis, ruling out the presence of coronary artery disease is very important before interpreting the images of the scans. SPECT-based cardiac imaging is one of the most commonly utilized imaging modalities to evaluate and manage common cardiac conditions. However, cardiac SPECT is not routinely performed for the evaluation of CS, given its low sensitivity and spatial resolution, especially compared to cardiac MRI and PET. In addition, the utilization of isotopes such as 201 TL results in an overall higher cumulative radiation exposure when compared to PET isotopes.[45]

ROLE OF CARDIAC 2-DEOXY-2-[FLUORINE-18]FLUORO-D-GLUCOSE POSITRON EMISSION TOMOGRAPHY (PET)

18F-FDG is a glucose analog actively taken up by inflammatory cells along with glucose. While glucose is metabolized further using the citric acid cycle, phosphorylated 18F-FDG remains inside the cells and can be imaged. MPI using 82Rb or 13N-Ammonia PET or a traditional SPECT is typically performed before 18F-FDG PET imaging to assess for inflammation.[46] Together, these two modalities help assess the stage and severity of the disease and provide useful therapeutic and prognostic information.

Ruling out the presence of coronary artery disease or its sequelae of CAD, such as a scar, is important before performing PET imaging for CS. Often these conditions lead to abnormalities in perfusion imaging which can cause erroneous interpretation of the scan. Patients with symptoms and risk factors with a high pretest probability of CAD should undergo screening with stress testing, cardiac CT with coronary angiography, or invasive coronary angiography. Similarly, the presence of other inflammatory conditions, such as myocarditis, cardiac involvement of rheumatoid arthritis, and so forth, depending on the clinical presentation of patients, should also be ruled out.

Preparation for Performing 18F-FDG PET

Adequate patient preparation, often achieved by combining various strategies that target different aspects of myocardial metabolism, is key in ensuring high specificity and positive predictive value of 18F-FDG PET. It usually begins 24 hours before the scheduled test time with dietary manipulation in the form of a high-fat and low-carbohydrate diet followed by a prolonged fasting period for at least 12 hours.[47] These steps promote myocardial consumption of free fatty acids over glucose as a primary source of energy and metabolism.

Once patients have undergone MPI imaging, 10 to 50 IU/kg of intravenous unfractionated heparin is injected about 15 minutes before 18F-FDG injections to promote lipolysis and increase the serum levels of free fatty acids. The protocol for preparation is typically modified and standardized for an institution and for the patients. Scans are obtained about 90 to 120 minutes after the injection of 18F-FDG. A low-dose CT scan is first performed for attenuation correction, followed by dedicated PET scanning of the myocardium and whole body.

Image Interpretation of 18F-FDG PET

After image processing and reconstruction have been satisfactorily performed, images are assessed for adequate myocardial suppression by ensuring there is either no visible myocardial 18F-FDG uptake or by ensuring that it is lower than that of the blood pool.

Table 3 illustrates the interpretation of the combination of findings on MPI and 18F-FDG PET imaging.[48] The likelihood of cardiac sarcoidosis is low in patients with a normal perfusion scan and no FDG uptake (**Fig. 2**). However, a mismatch of defects on perfusion imaging from those in 18F-FDG PET indicated progressive disease with active inflammation. Advanced disease with

A   B

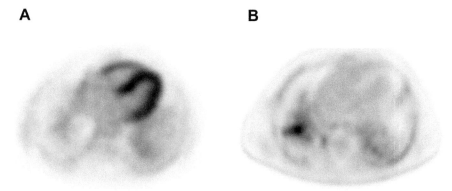

Fig. 2. A 57-year-old female patient with dyspnea on exertion and chest discomfort on exertion, who has biopsy proven pulmonary sarcoidosis, referred for 8F-FDG PET. Image A shows normal myocardial perfusion imaging performed using Rb-82 PET myocardial perfusion imaging. Image B depicts 18F-FDG PET scan showing no uptake of 18F-FDG, indicating absence of cardiac involvement by sarcoidosis.

resulting fibrosis may manifest as severe perfusion defects without uptake of 18F-FDG, whereas early disease manifests as normal MPI with abnormal 18F-FDG uptake on the metabolic scan (**Fig. 3**). Mild resting perfusion defects without 18F-FDG uptake may still indicate the presence of cardiac sarcoidosis but without active inflammation.[48,49]

The mere presence of focal 18F-FDG uptake is not a specific marker of CS. Likewise, the presence of isolated mild-intensity lateral wall uptake is a non-specific finding and does not indicate the presence of CS. Similarly, inadequately prepared patients can have a diffuse 18F-FDG uptake (**Fig. 4**), often necessitating repeating the 18F-FDG PET part of the study after appropriate patient preparation. Resting perfusion defects in CS result from compression of coronary arterioles in the microvascular beds due to active inflammation or granuloma formation or from the replacement of myocardium with fibrous tissue.[50,51]

The postulated sensitivity and specificity of 18F-FDG PET are derived from several meta-analyses and systematic reviews, which in turn have pooled data from various small-scale studies, not devoid of bias, lack of standard reference, and differing protocols.[49–52] The sensitivity and specificity of 18F-FDG PET in detecting CS among all these studies range between 81%–89% and 78%–83%, respectively.

Therapeutic and Prognostic Value of 18F-FDG PET

In addition to diagnostic capabilities, 18F-FDG PET demonstrates significant prognostic and therapeutic value. In fact, it is the preferred modality to assess response to therapy. Quantitative analysis entails the assessment of the concentration of radioactive tracer in a region of interest (measured in Bq/mL) corrected for the injected dose and the patient's weight, represented as SUVmax.[53]

A   B

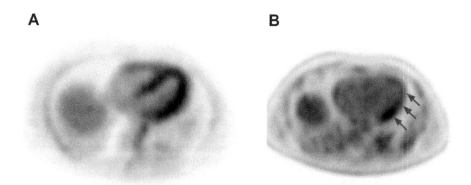

Fig. 3. A 63-year-old male with recurrent atrial tachyarrhythmia, congestive heart failure, and skin lesions suspicious for sarcoidosis is referred for 18F-FDG PET scan to rule out cardiac sarcoidosis. Image A depicts a Rb-82 based PET myocardial perfusion imaging with relatively normal perfusion. Image B shows 18F-FDG uptake in the lateral wall extending from the basal segments to the apical segments (depicted with *arrows*).

A   **B**

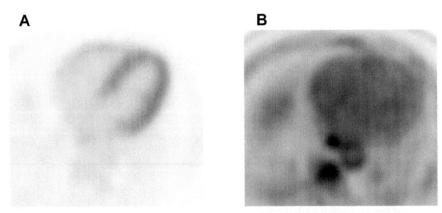

Fig. 4. A 70-year-old female patient who was referred from an outside hospital for ^{18}F-FDG PET scan for the assessment of cardiac sarcoidosis. Image A shows a normal Rb-82 PET myocardial perfusion but upon patient performing ^{18}F-FDG scan (*B*), there is evidence of ^{18}F-FDG in the blood pool. The patient later admitted to not complying with dietary recommendations.

Several quantitative metrics have been developed to quantify the degree of myocardial involvement, which can be followed in time to assess response to therapy.[54,55] Reduction in the extent and intensity of inflammation on serial PET in response to immunosuppressive therapy has been associated with improved LV systolic function. However, data on the correlation of quantitative assessment with long-term outcomes are currently lacking.

Certain features on 18F-FDG PET represent high-risk findings and may help identify patients at an elevated risk of adverse clinical outcomes who may benefit from more careful surveillance and aggressive therapeutic measures. Pathologic RV uptake of 18F-FDG (**Fig. 5**) has been identified as one of the strongest predictors for mortality, ventricular tachyarrhythmia, and reduction in LVEF, with some studies showing almost 5-fold increased risk of adverse cardiac events.[56,57] In a study by Blankenstein and colleagues, 118 patients without a history of coronary artery disease were referred for PET imaging for the evaluation of known or suspected cardiac sarcoidosis. 18F-FDG was used to assess inflammation, and rubidium-82 was used to evaluate perfusion defects. PET findings were classified as normal, positive perfusion defect or FDG, and positive perfusion defect and FDG. Median follow-up was 1.5 years, and adverse events were defined as either sustained ventricular tachycardia or all-cause mortality. The authors reported annualized event rates of 7.3%, 18.4%, and 31.9% for patients with normal perfusion and no FDG uptake or diffuse FDG uptake, abnormal perfusion or focal FDG uptake, and abnormal perfusion and focal FDG uptake, respectively. Additionally, of the 11 patients with focal RV FDG uptake, 8 patients

experienced an adverse event corresponding to an annualized event rate of 55.2%, again underscoring the importance of considering focal FDG uptake in the RV as a poor prognostic indicator.[57] However, it is important to note that the presence of perfusion-metabolism mismatch itself predicts a higher risk of adverse cardiovascular events.[58] Active inflammation persisting on serial 18F-FDG PET scans is strongly associated with progressive disease, ultimately leading to worsening of LV systolic function along with independent poor long-term outcomes such as the recurrence of VT, HF

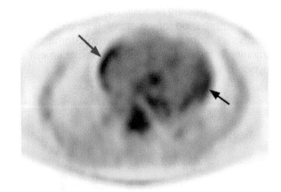

Fig. 5. A 42-year-old male who presented with new onset ventricular tachycardia that did not respond to amiodarone or procainamide boluses and ultimately required synchronized cardioversion for hemodynamic instability. Cardiac MRI done for evaluation for new onset cardiomyopathy showed mid-myocardial late gadolinium enhancement of the basal infero-septum (see **Fig. 6**) raising suspicion for cardiac sarcoidosis. An ^{18}F-FDG PET scan thereafter showed patchy uptake of ^{8}F-FDG in the lateral wall and right ventricle (see Fig. 5). The (*arrows*) show the areas of uptake.

hospitalization, and increased overall mortality.[59] A 20-fold increased risk of major adverse cardiovascular events was noted among patients considered non-responders to immunosuppressive therapies at follow-up.[59]

In a recent study by Patel and colleagues, the authors tried to determine what clinical and imaging characteristics were predictive of adverse outcomes in patients with known or suspected cardiac sarcoidosis that was not on immunosuppressant therapy. PET results can be confounded by immunosuppressant therapy, and previous studies have included patients on immunosuppressant therapy, which is why the authors chose to focus on this subgroup of patients. They retrospectively analyzed 197 patients who underwent PET imaging to evaluate known or suspected cardiac sarcoidosis. The primary outcome was time to ventricular arrhythmia [VT/VF] or death, and the median follow-up was 531 days. They found that LVEF, a history of VT/VF, and summed rest score [SRS] were predictors of the primary endpoint [$P < .05$], whereas quantitative and qualitative measures of FDG uptake did not predict clinical events. As measured on quantitative analysis, the extent and amount of inflammation are necessary to understand the overall outcomes, identify patients who may benefit from early aggressive strategies, and refer them to advanced HF specialists.[60]

ROLE OF CARDIAC MAGNETIC RESONANCE IMAGING

Cardiac MRI is considered an indispensable tool for the evaluation of CS. It is often the first imaging modality to screen patients with sarcoidosis for cardiac involvement. With its superior resolution and unique ability to image myocardial edema, perfusion abnormalities, and fibrosis, it has become an indispensable tool in diagnosing and managing CS. In addition, it also allows for the evaluation of myocardial geometry and wall motion accurately. The lack of radiation combined with the relatively lower risk of gadolinium-associated side effects makes MRI more appealing than other imaging techniques. However, certain implants and devices in the body, especially when composed of metals, may preclude the performance of the scan, given the interaction within the magnetic field. While the use of gadolinium-based agents is safe in patients with chronic kidney disease when the estimated glomerular filtration rate (eGFR) > 30 mL/min/1.73 m2, among patients with eGFR less than 30 mL/min/1.73 m2 or on hemodialysis, newer agents may be considered keeping in mind the risk of systemic nephrogenic fibrosis.[61]

Cardiac Magnetic Resonance Imaging Acquisition for the Evaluation of Cardiac Sarcoidosis

Imaging protocols using cMRI are typically modified for each patient and their respective clinical presentation. However, most protocols consist of cine images along multiple planes, T2-weighted imaging to evaluate for myocardial edema, and LGE imaging to assess the presence of fibrosis.[46] In addition, T1 and T2 mapping is sometimes added to the sequences to detect focal enhancement and suggest the presence of edema/inflammation.[46]

Cine cMRI allows taking pictures of the entire heart in the prescribed stacks along the long and short axes, delineating the structure and function of the myocardium in the highest resolution. Short Tau Inversion Recovery methods used in T2-weighted (T2-STIR) images detect the presence of free water in the myocardium, thus indirectly assessing the presence, degree, and location of edema and inflammation. LGE imaging employs saturation recovery techniques to evaluate areas of the myocardium with the expanded extracellular matrix as a sequela of infiltration and fibrosis. Parametric T1 and T2 mapping allows the quantitative measurement of tissue affected by inflammation, edema, and fibrosis. Though T1 is strongly sensitive to abnormal myocardium, it is non-specific to differentiate myocardial fibrosis or edema. On the other hand, T2 mapping is more water sensitive. A combination of these two imaging methods helps to identify either inflammatory (raised native T2) or fibrotic (normal native T2) changes in the myocardium.[62]

Image Interpretation of Cardiac Magnetic Resonance Imaging

While the presence of focal LGE in mid-myocardial or sub-epicardial patterns in the basal, septal, and lateral walls is the most common finding in patients with CS (**Fig. 6**),[63,64] differing patterns and extent of LGE have been reported. LGE does not always suggest a diagnosis of sarcoidosis, as a similar pattern can often be found in several other inflammatory conditions, particularly myocarditis. In a recent study by Poyhonen and colleagues that compared 18 patients with giant cell myocarditis [GCM] to a cohort consisting of patients with cardiac sarcoidosis that were matched for age, sex, LV EF, and presenting cardiac manifestations, the authors found that the qualitative cMRI findings including LGE distribution were indistinguishable between the two entities, including the "hook sign" seen in cardiac sarcoidosis even though myocardial inflammation

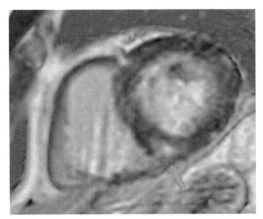

Fig. 6. A 42-year-old male who presented with new onset ventricular tachycardia that did not respond to amiodarone or procainamide boluses and ultimately required synchronized cardioversion for hemodynamic instability. Cardiac MRI done for evaluation for new onset cardiomyopathy showed mid-myocardial late gadolinium enhancement of the basal infero-septum (see Fig. 6) raising suspicion for cardiac sarcoidosis. An ¹⁸F-FDG PET scan thereafter showed patchy uptake of ⁸F-FDG in the lateral wall and right ventricle (see **Fig. 5**; image B). The (arrows) shows an areas of LGE.

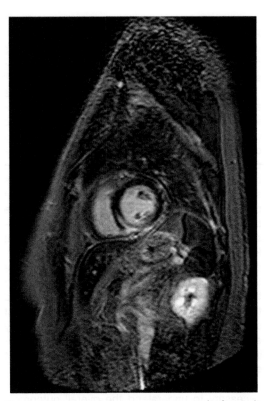

Fig. 7. LGE (late gadolinium enhancement) of an individual with cardiac sarcoidosis few years apart showing the progression of LGE.

was more acute in the giant cell myocarditis group. They found LV size and total LGE mass were lower in the GCM cohort.[65]

Features seen in the late stages of the disease, such as septal thinning and regional motion abnormalities, are better appreciated in cine images. T2-weighted images may show evidence of myocardial edema and/or inflammation, but there is significant overlap with other inflammatory conditions. T2-weighted imaging can sometimes be limited in application due to the relatively low signal-to-noise ratio and vulnerability of the MRI sequence to artifacts. Native T1 imaging and assessment of extracellular volume (ECV) also add to the diagnostic sensitivity of the test and help identify abnormal regions of the myocardium.[65]

If the diagnosis remains elusive, distinguishing CS from myocarditis by cMRI can also be aided by follow-up cMRI imaging in 4 to 5 months. **Figs. 7** and **8** demonstrate the progression of late gadolinium enhancement in a patient with cardiac sarcoidosis a few years apart. The cMRI findings in acute myocarditis tend to be dynamic, while those in sarcoid are less likely to change over time. Other imaging features that favor cardiac sarcoid are the presence of LGE in the basal septum, wall motion abnormalities in segments with abundant LGE, and contiguous LGE that, when viewed along the long axis of the left

ventricle, includes epicardial, mid-myocardial, and endocardial portions.[65]

The ideal diagnostic approach entails interpreting all the above features in patients with high clinical suspicion. A meta-analysis of several studies assessing the accuracy of cMRI in diagnosing CS has shown improved detection when different imaging findings such as LGE, T2-weighted imaging, and tissue mapping are combined.[52] Overall, cMRI is considered more sensitive than 18F-FDG PET in diagnosing CS, with sensitivity from a large meta-analysis being around 95% (vs 84% for 18F-FDG PET; $P = .002$). However, the specificity was reported to be similar to 18F-FDG PET, at 85%. The specificity for 18F-FDG PET was 82% ($P = .85$).[52]

Therapeutic and Prognostic Value of Cardiac Magnetic Resonance Imaging

Unlike 18F-FDG PET, cMRI has a limited role in guiding response to therapy. While T2-weighted imaging can help identify areas of possible inflammation, this can be a non-specific finding and hard to follow up. Quantitative assessment using tissue mapping may offer insights into objective improvement and response to therapy but currently lacks evidence.

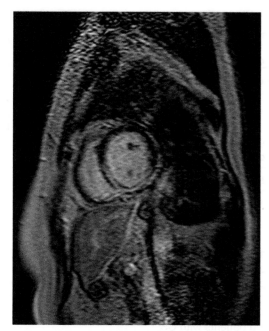

Fig. 8. LGE (late gadolinium enhancement) of an individual with cardiac sarcoidosis few years apart showing the progression of LGE.

Several studies have demonstrated the powerful prognostic capabilities of LGE in patients with CS. In a meta-analysis of 694 patients by Hulten and colleagues presence of LGE was associated with a significantly increased risk of cardiovascular and all-cause mortality and ventricular arrhythmias compared to patients without evidence of LGE.[66] LGE among a cohort of 155 patients was identified as an independent risk factor for mortality, aborted death, and appropriate implantable cardioverter defibrillator (ICD) discharge.[67] Studies on patients with CS have shown higher extracellular volume, higher myocardial native T1 and T2, and lower ventricular longitudinal strain in cMRI, with a significant reduction of native T1 and T2 in the patients after treatment. The finding establishes the potential role of cMRI for the follow-up of patients with CS on treatment.[62]

Athwal and colleagues showed that among a cohort of 504 patients with histologically confirmed CS, certain specific LGE patterns, such as RV and multifocal involvement, conferred a higher risk regardless of LVEF or quantified LGE burden.[68] The study included patients from multiple different ethnic groups. The patients were divided into various cMRI phenotypes based on LGE findings. They categorized patients into a "pathology-frequent" LGE group which included LV subepicardial, LV multifocal, septal, and RV free wall involvement, and a "pathology-rare" group which included no myocardial LGE, isolated mid myocardial LGE, isolated LV subendocardial involvement and the absence of septal involvement. The pathology frequent LGE group (n = 103; 20.4%) was associated with a high risk of arrhythmic events. Among this group (n = 103), 28.2% were females, 71.8% were males, 81.6% were white, and 14.6% were black. According to ethnicity, most patients (99%) were non-Hispanic or Latino.[68]

Interestingly, some studies show differences in presenting symptoms, cardiac involvement in cMRI, and prognosis in patients with suspected CS based on their demographic characteristics. For example, Kalra and colleagues showed no difference in cardiac involvement based on the diagnostic criteria for CS in male and female patients. Also, the long-term incidence of all-cause death or significant ventricular arrhythmia was the same in male and female patients.[69] Another study by Velangi and colleagues showed that patients with sarcoidosis, RV systolic dysfunction, and RV LGE had distinct prognostic values. RV systolic dysfunction (68.6% white, 25.7% black) was independently associated with all-cause death. RV LGE (87.5% white, 6.3% black) was independently associated with sudden cardiac death or significant ventricular arrhythmia.[70] These findings can help study CS in patients according to their sex, race, and ethnicity to help diagnose and manage them accordingly.

Patients with CS presenting with the atrioventricular block are at risk for life-threatening ventricular arrhythmias and sudden cardiac death. Also, they are at risk of developing heart failure. Cardiac MRI is an effective screening tool for patients with heart block, on a temporary pacemaker, for the early detection of CS.[71] Studies on complete heart block patients with CS who has MRI conditional pacemaker has also shown the diagnostic accuracy of cMRI.[72]

While the 2017 American Heart Association/American College of Cardiology/Heart Rhythm Society (AHA/ACC/HRS) guideline for the management of patients with ventricular arrhythmias and the prevention of sudden cardiac death give a class IIa indication for the implantation of ICD in patients with CS and LVEF greater than 35% if there is evidence of "extensive LGE" on cMRI, the exact definition of extensive LGE is not yet clear.[73]

COMBINED MAGNETIC RESONANCE IMAGING AND 18F-FDG PET

Retrospective analysis of various studies has shown cMRI to be more sensitive but less specific than FDG-PET in predicting adverse events in

Table 4
Diagnostic interpretation of combined cardiac MRI and ^{18}F-FDG PET testing

Interpretation	Findings on cMRI	Findings on ^{18}F-FDG PET
Active disease with the presence of scar and inflammation[a]	Presence of LGE	^{18}F-FDG uptake noted
Scar without active inflammation (inactive disease)	Presence of LGE	No ^{18}F-FDG PET uptake noted
Normal (no disease)	Absence of LGE	Absence of ^{18}F-FDG PET uptake
Early disease/False positive	Absence of LGE	^{18}F-FDG uptake noted

Abbreviations: 18F-FDG-PET, Positron emission tomography with 2-deoxy-2-[fluorine-18] fluoro- D-glucose; cMRI, cardiac magnetic resonance imaging; LGE, late gadolinium enhancement.
[a] The patterns of LGE (on cMRI) and ^{18}F-FDG uptake (on ^{18}F-FDG PET) usually align.
Data from Refs.[76–78]

patients with CS.[74] One systematic review and meta-analysis by Aitken and colleagues found that LGE at cMRI and FDG-PET were both associated with adverse cardiac events. However, cardiac MRI might have a higher prognostic value.[75] By combining cardiac MRI and 18F-FDG PET, patients can be segregated into four groups depending on the presence or absence of both LGE on cMRI and 18F-FDG on the PET scan. **Table 4** illustrates the interpretation when combining both modalities. While this has yet to be well validated in large-scale studies, several small-scale studies have shown superior benefits of combined modalities over either alone.[76–78] Combined abnormalities noted on both scans were significantly superior in predicting major adverse cardiovascular events than abnormalities on a single modality alone.[76,78] In addition, the sensitivity and specificity of combined approaches were noted to be far superior to either modality. These modalities also boasted lower cumulative radiation exposure. Large-scale studies are needed to validate these results, evaluate the long-term outcomes, and assess response with therapy.

SUMMARY

This review illustrates the use of different imaging tools for the diagnosis of CS. The advantages and limitations of various imaging modalities have been discussed. The role of cardiac imaging in the evaluation CS is still an emerging area necessitating further study. More information is required to determine how to best incorporate findings from different imaging modalities in establishing a diagnosis of CS. Additionally, more specific guidelines are needed on the optimal use of these imaging modalities to monitor patients on the timeline of follow-up imaging, and on the duration of treatment. In the future, multicenter randomized studies may be able to help better

answer these questions. Timely diagnosis of CS and its complications, if any, will prompt appropriate treatment and increase the likelihood of positive outcomes. For this reason, the application of advanced imaging is an integral part in managing patients with CS.

CLINICS CARE POINTS

- Cardiac sarcoid remains a difficult disease to diagnose clinically
- The concurrent use of CMR and PET provides the highest sensitivity for the diagnosis of cardiac sarcoid

DISCLOSURE

None of the authors have anything to disclose.

REFERENCES

1. Kowalska M, Niewiadomska E, Zejda JE. Epidemiology of sarcoidosis recorded in 2006-2010 in the Silesian voivodeship on the basis of routine medical reporting. Ann Agric Environ Med 2014;21(1):55–8.
2. Selroos O. The frequency, clinical picture and prognosis of pulmonary sarcoidosis in Finland. Acta Med Scand Suppl 1969;503:3–73.
3. Geraint DJ. Pioneers of sarcoidosis: Jonathan Hutchinson (1828-1913). Sarcoidosis Vasc Diffuse Lung Dis. Jun 2002;19(2):120.
4. James DG, Sharma OP. From Hutchinson to now: a historical glimpse. Curr Opin Pulm Med. Sep 2002; 8(5):416–23.
5. Pour-Ghaz I, Kayali S, Abutineh I, et al. Cardiac Sarcoidosis: Pathophysiology, Diagnosis, and Management. Hearts 2021;2(2):234–50.

6. Ayoub C, Pena E, Ohira H, et al. Advanced imaging of cardiac sarcoidosis. Curr Cardiol Rep 2015;17(4):1–2.

7. Brito-Zerón P, Kostov B, Superville D, et al. Geoepidemiological big data approach to sarcoidosis: geographical and ethnic determinants. Clin Exp Rheumatol 2019;37(6):1052–64.

8. Spagnolo P, Rossi G, Trisolini R, et al. Pulmonary sarcoidosis. Lancet Respir Med 2018;6(5):389–402.

9. Kusano KF, Satomi K. Diagnosis and treatment of cardiac sarcoidosis. Heart 2016;102(3):184–90.

10. Sharma A, Okada DR, Yacoub H, et al. Diagnosis of cardiac sarcoidosis: an era of paradigm shift. Ann Nucl Med 2020;34(2):87–93.

11. Mirsaeidi M, Machado RF, Schraufnagel D, et al. Racial difference in sarcoidosis mortality in the United States. Chest 2015;147(2):438–49.

12. Martusewicz-Boros MM, Boros PW, Wiatr E, et al. Cardiac Sarcoidosis: Is it More Common in Men? Lung 2016;194(1):61–6.

13. Cheong BY, Muthupillai R, Nemeth M, et al. The utility of delayed-enhancement magnetic resonance imaging for identifying nonischemic myocardial fibrosis in asymptomatic patients with biopsy-proven systemic sarcoidosis. Sarcoidosis Vasc Diffuse Lung Dis 2009;26(1):39–46.

14. Kandolin R, Lehtonen J, Graner M, et al. Diagnosing isolated cardiac sarcoidosis. J Intern Med 2011;270(5):461–8.

15. Birnie DH, Sauer WH, Bogun F, et al. HRS expert consensus statement on the diagnosis and management of arrhythmias associated with cardiac sarcoidosis. Heart Rhythm 2014;11(7):1305–23.

16. Terasaki F, Azuma A, Anzai T, et al. JCS 2016 Guideline on Diagnosis and Treatment of Cardiac Sarcoidosis - Digest Version. Circ J 2019;83(11):2329–88.

17. Markatis E, Afthinos A, Antonakis E, et al. Cardiac sarcoidosis: diagnosis and management. Rev Cardiovasc Med 2020;21(3):321–38.

18. Uusimaa P, Ylitalo K, Anttonen O, et al. Ventricular tachyarrhythmia as a primary presentation of sarcoidosis. Europace 2008;10(6):760–6.

19. Johns CJ, Michele TM. The clinical management of sarcoidosis. A 50-year experience at the Johns Hopkins Hospital. Medicine (Baltim) 1999;78(2):65–111.

20. Sharma OP, Maheshwari A, Thaker K. Myocardial sarcoidosis. Chest 1993;103(1):253–8.

21. Yazaki Y, Isobe M, Hiroe M, et al. Prognostic determinants of long-term survival in Japanese patients with cardiac sarcoidosis treated with prednisone. Am J Cardiol 2001;88(9):1006–10.

22. Asimaki A, Tandri H, Duffy ER, et al. Altered desmosomal proteins in granulomatous myocarditis and potential pathogenic links to arrhythmogenic right ventricular cardiomyopathy. Circ Arrhythm Electrophysiol 2011;4(5):743–52.

23. Trivieri MG, Spagnolo P, Birnie D, et al. Challenges in cardiac and pulmonary sarcoidosis: JACC state-of-the-art review. J Am Coll Cardiol 2020;76(16):1878–901.

24. Manabe O, Oyama-Manabe N, Aikawa T, et al. Advances in Diagnostic Imaging for Cardiac Sarcoidosis. J Clin Med 2021;10(24):5808.

25. Jeny F, Bernaudin JF, Aubart FC, et al. Diagnosis issues in sarcoidosis. Respiratory Medicine and Research 2020;77:37–45.

26. Divakaran S, Stewart GC, Lakdawala NK, et al. Diagnostic accuracy of advanced imaging in cardiac sarcoidosis: an imaging-histologic correlation study in patients undergoing cardiac transplantation. Circulation: Cardiovascular Imaging 2019;12(6):e008975.

27. Hulten E, Aslam S, Osborne M, et al. Cardiac sarcoidosis-state of the art review. Cardiovasc Diagn Ther 2016;6(1):50–63.

28. Casal A, Suárez-Antelo J, Soto-Feijóo R, et al. Sarcoidosis. Disease progression based on radiological and functional course:Predictive factors. Heart Lung 2022;56:62–9.

29. Baughman Robert P, Judson Marc A. Relapses of sarcoidosis: what are they and can we predict who will get them? European Respiratory Journal Feb 2014;43(2):337–9.

30. Rosario KF, Brezitski K, Arps K, et al. Cardiac Sarcoidosis: Current Approaches to Diagnosis and Management. Curr Allergy Asthma Rep 2022;1–2.

31. Wand AL, Chrispin J, Saad E, et al. Current state and future directions of multimodality imaging in cardiac sarcoidosis. Frontiers in Cardiovascular Medicine 2021;2275.

32. Solmaz H, Ozdogan O. Left atrial phasic volumes and functions changes in asymptomatic patients with sarcoidosis: evaluation by three-dimensional echocardiography. Acta Cardiol 2022;1–9.

33. Houston BA, Mukherjee M. Cardiac sarcoidosis: clinical manifestations, imaging characteristics, and therapeutic approach. Clin Med Insights Cardiol 2014;8(Suppl 1):31–7.

34. Di Stefano C, Bruno G, Arciniegas Calle MC, et al. Diagnostic and predictive value of speckle tracking echocardiography in cardiac sarcoidosis. BMC Cardiovasc Disord 2020;20:21.

35. Cabuk AK, Cabuk G. Real-time three-dimensional echocardiography for detection of cardiac sarcoidosis in the early stage: a cross-sectional single-centre study. Acta Cardiol 2022;1–9.

36. Lo Gullo A, Rodríguez-Carrio J, Gallizzi R, et al. Speckle tracking echocardiography as a new diagnostic tool for an assessment of cardiovascular disease in rheumatic patients. Prog Cardiovasc Dis 2020;63(3):327–40.

37. Albakaa NK, Sato K, Iida N, et al. Association between right ventricular longitudinal strain and cardiovascular events in patients with cardiac sarcoidosis. J Cardiol 2022;80(6):549–56.

38. Surasi DS, Manapragada PP, Lloyd SG, et al. Role of multimodality imaging including thallium-201 myocardial perfusion imaging in the diagnosis and monitoring of treatment response in cardiac sarcoidosis. J Nucl Cardiol 2014;21:849–52.

39. Eguchi M, Tsuchihashi K, Hotta D, et al. Technetium-99m sestamibi/tetrofosmin myocardial perfusion scanning in cardiac and noncardiac sarcoidosis. Cardiology 2000;94:193–9.

40. Fields CL, Ossorio MA, Roy TM, et al. Thallium-201 scintigraphy in the diagnosis and management of myocardial sarcoidosis. South Med J 1990;83(3):339–42.

41. Silberstein EB, DeVries DF. Reverse redistribution phenomenon in thallium-201 stress tests: angiographic correlation and clinical significance. J Nucl Med 1985;26:707–10.

42. Okayama K, Kurata C, Tawarahara K, et al. Diagnostic and prognostic value of myocardial scintigraphy with thallium-201 and gallium-67 in cardiac sarcoidosis. Chest 1995;107(2):330–4.

43. Tamaki N, Yoshinaga K. Novel iodinated tracers, MIBG and BMIPP for nuclear cardiology. J Nucl Cardiol 2011;18(1):135–43.

44. Campisi R, Merani MF, Marina MI. BMIPP SPECT in cardiac sarcoidosis: a marker of risk? J Nucl Cardiol 2021;28(3):930–5.

45. Desiderio MC, Lundbye JB, Baker WL, et al. Current Status of Patient Radiation Exposure of Cardiac Positron Emission Tomography and Single-Photon Emission Computed Tomographic Myocardial Perfusion Imaging: A Report From the Intersocietal Accreditation Commission Database. Circulation: Cardiovascular Imaging 2018;11(12):e007565.

46. Slart RHJA, Glaudemans AWJM, Lancellotti P, et al. A joint procedural position statement on imaging in cardiac sarcoidosis: from the Cardiovascular and Inflammation & Infection Committees of the European Association of Nuclear Medicine, the European Association of Cardiovascular Imaging, and the American Society of Nuclear Cardiology. J Nucl Cardiol 2018;25(1):298–319.

47. Osborne MT, Hulten EA, Murthy VL, et al. Patient preparation for cardiac fluorine-18 fluorodeoxyglucose positron emission tomography imaging of inflammation. J Nucl Cardiol 2017;24:86–99.

48. Blankstein R, Waller AH. Evaluation of known or suspected cardiac sarcoidosis. Circ Cardiovasc Imaging 2016;9:e000867.

49. Youssef G, Leung E, Mylonas I, et al. The use of 18F-FDG PET in the diagnosis of cardiac sarcoidosis: a systematic review and metaanalysis including the Ontario experience. J Nucl Med 2012;53(2):241–8.

50. Kim SJ, Pak K, Kim K. Diagnostic performance of F-18 FDG PET for detection of cardiac sarcoidosis; A systematic review and meta-analysis. J Nucl Cardiol 2020;27(6):2103–15.

51. Tang R, Wang JTY, Wang L, et al. Impact of patient preparation on the diagnostic performance of 18F-FDG PET in cardiac sarcoidosis: a systematic review and meta-analysis. Clin Nucl Med 2016;41(7):e327–39.

52. Aitken M, Chan MV, Urzua Fresno C, et al. Diagnostic Accuracy of Cardiac MRI versus FDG PET for Cardiac Sarcoidosis: A Systematic Review and Meta-Analysis. Radiology 2022;213170.

53. Okumura W, Iwasaki T, Toyama T, et al. Usefulness of fasting 18F-FDG PET in identification of cardiac sarcoidosis. J Nucl Med 2004;45:1989–98.

54. Ahmadian A, Pawar S, Govender P, et al. The response of FDG uptake to immunosuppressive treatment on FDG PET/CT imaging for cardiac sarcoidosis. J Nucl Cardiol 2017;24:413–24.

55. Waller AH, Blankstein R. Quantifying myocardial inflammation using F18-fluorodeoxyglucose positron emission tomography in cardiac sarcoidosis. J Nucl Cardiol 2014;21:940–3.

56. Tuominen H, Haarala A, Tikkakoski A, et al. FDG-PET in possible cardiac sarcoidosis: Right ventricular uptake and high total cardiac metabolic activity predict cardiovascular events. J Nucl Cardiol 2021;28(1):199–205.

57. Blankstein R, Osborne M, Naya M, et al. Cardiac positron emission tomography enhances prognostic assessments of patients with suspected cardiac sarcoidosis. J Am Coll Cardiol 2014;63:329–36.

58. Sperry BW, Tamarappoo BK, Oldan JD, et al. Prognostic impact of extent, severity, and heterogeneity of abnormalities on (18)F-FDG PET scans for suspected cardiac sarcoidosis. JACC Cardiovasc Imaging 2018;11:336–45.

59. Muser D, Santangeli P, Castro SA, et al. Prognostic role of serial quantitative evaluation of 18F-fluorodeoxyglucose uptake by PET/CT in patients with cardiac sarcoidosis presenting with ventricular tachycardia. Eur J Nucl Med Mol Imaging 2018;45:1394–404.

60. Patel VN, Pieper JA, Poitrasson-Rivière A, et al. The prognostic value of positron emission tomography in the evaluation of suspected cardiac sarcoidosis. J Nucl Cardiol 2022;29(5):2460–70.

61. Schieda N, Blaichman JI, Costa AF, et al. Gadolinium-Based Contrast Agents in Kidney Disease: A Comprehensive Review and Clinical Practice Guideline Issued by the Canadian Association of Radiologists. Canadian Journal of Kidney Health and Disease 2018;5. https://doi.org/10.1177/2054358118778573.

62. Puntmann VO, Isted A, Hinojar R, et al. T1 and T2 mapping in recognition of early cardiac involvement in systemic sarcoidosis. Radiology 2017;285(1):63–72.

63. Patel MR, Cawley PJ, Heitner JF, et al. Detection of myocardial damage in patients with sarcoidosis. Circulation 2009;120:1969–77.

64. Ichinose A, Otani H, Oikawa M, et al. MRI of cardiac sarcoidosis: basal and subepicardial localization of myocardial lesions and their effect on left ventricular function. AJR 2008;191:862–9.

65. Pöyhönen Pauli, Nordenswan Hanna-Kaisa, Lehtonen Jukka, et al. Cardiac magnetic resonance in giant cell myocarditis: a matched comparison with cardiac sarcoidosis. European Heart Journal - Cardiovascular Imaging 2023;24(4):404–12.

66. Hulten E, Agarwal V, Cahill M, et al. Presence of late gadolinium enhancement by cardiac magnetic resonance among patients with suspected cardiac sarcoidosis is associated with adverse cardiovascular prognosis: a systematic review and meta-analysis. Circulation: Cardiovascular Imaging 2016;9(9):e005001.

67. Greulich S, Deluigi CC, Gloekler S, et al. CMR imaging predicts death and other adverse events in suspected cardiac sarcoidosis. JACC Cardiovasc Imaging 2013;6:501–11.

68. Athwal PSS, Chhikara S, Ismail MF, et al. Cardiovascular Magnetic Resonance Imaging Phenotypes and Long-term Outcomes in Patients With Suspected Cardiac Sarcoidosis. JAMA Cardiol 2022;7(10):1057–66.

69. Kalra R, Malik S, Chen KA, et al. Sex Differences in Patients With Suspected Cardiac Sarcoidosis Assessed by Cardiovascular Magnetic Resonance Imaging. Circ Arrhythm Electrophysiol 2021;14(9):e009966.

70. Velangi PS, Chen KA, Kazmirczak F, et al. Right Ventricular Abnormalities on Cardiovascular Magnetic Resonance Imaging in Patients With Sarcoidosis. JACC Cardiovasc Imaging 2020;13(6):1395–405.

71. Vuorinen AM, Lehtonen J, Pakarinen S, et al. Cardiac Magnetic Resonance Imaging-Based Screening for Cardiac Sarcoidosis in Patients With Atrioventricular Block Requiring Temporary Pacing. J Am Heart Assoc 2022;11(11):e024257.

72. Orii M, Tanimoto T, Ota S, et al. Diagnostic accuracy of cardiac magnetic resonance imaging for cardiac sarcoidosis in complete heart block patients implanted with magnetic resonance-conditional pacemaker. J Cardiol 2020;76(2):191–7.

73. Al-Khatib SM, Stevenson WG, Ackerman MJ, et al. 2017 AHA/ACC/HRS guideline for management of patients with ventricular arrhythmias and the prevention of sudden cardiac death: a report of the American College of Cardiology/American Heart Association task force on clinical practice guidelines and the Heart Rhythm Society. Circulation 2018;138(13):e272–391.

74. Adhaduk M, Paudel B, Khalid MU, et al. Comparison of cardiac magnetic resonance imaging and fluorodeoxyglucose positron emission tomography in the assessment of cardiac sarcoidosis: Meta-analysis and systematic review. J Nucl Cardiol 2022. https://doi.org/10.1007/s12350-022-03129-8.

75. Aitken M, Davidson M, Chan MV, et al. Prognostic Value of Cardiac MRI and FDG PET in Cardiac Sarcoidosis: A Systematic Review and Meta-Analysis. Radiology 2023;307(2):e222483.

76. Dweck MR, Abgral R, Trivieri MG, et al. Hybrid magnetic resonance imaging and positron emission tomography with fluorodeoxyglucose to diagnose active cardiac sarcoidosis. JACC Cardiovasc Imaging 2017;11:94.

77. Wicks EC, Menezes LJ, Barnes A, et al. Diagnostic accuracy and prognostic value of simultaneous hybrid 18F-fluorodeoxyglucose positron emission tomography/magnetic resonance imaging in cardiac sarcoidosis. Eur Heart J Cardiovasc Imaging 2018;19:757–67.

78. Cheung E, Ahmad S, Aitken M, et al. Combined simultaneous FDG-PET/MRI with T1 and T2 mapping as an imaging biomarker for the diagnosis and prognosis of suspected cardiac sarcoidosis. European journal of hybrid imaging 2021;5(1):1–8.

Multimodality Imaging in Aortic Stenosis
Beyond the Valve - Focusing on the Myocardium

Safwan Gaznabi, MD[a,b], Jeirym Miranda, MD[a,c], Daniel Lorenzatti, MD[a],
Pamela Piña, MD[a,d], Senthil S. Balasubramanian, MD[b], Darshi Desai, MD[e],
Aditya Desai, MD[e], Edwin C. Ho, MD[a], Andrea Scotti, MD[a],
Carlos A. Gongora, MD[a], Aldo L. Schenone, MD[a], Mario J. Garcia, MD[a],
Azeem Latib, MD[a], Purvi Parwani, MBBS, MPH[f], Leandro Slipczuk, MD, PhD[a,*]

KEYWORDS

- Aortic stenosis • Low flow low gradient • Discordant • Asymptomatic • Global longitudinal strain
- Fibrosis • Myocardium

KEY POINTS

- Aortic stenosis is a complex, multifaceted disease leading to myocardial remodeling and ultimately to heart failure or sudden death.
- Traditional focus is shifting from the valve alone to integrate the myocardium through the evaluation of subclinical left ventricle remodeling and myocardial fibrosis to identify the best timing for aortic valve replacement (AVR).
- Echocardiography-driven cardiac damage and myocardial deformation parameters (global longitudinal strain and left atrium strain) are independently associated with outcomes pre- and post-AVR.
- Cardiovascular magnetic resonance evaluation can predict outcomes based on the evaluation of reversible interstitial fibrosis (increased T1/ extracellular volume) and irreversible replacement fibrosis (late gadolinium enhancement).
- Cardiac computed tomography allows for the evaluation of myocardial deformation, interstitial fibrosis, and advanced valve characterization.

BEYOND A VALVE-FOCUSED ASSESSMENT AND MANAGEMENT OF AORTIC STENOSIS

Aortic stenosis (AS) is a progressive and potentially fatal disease that leads to an increased afterload of the left ventricle (LV), subsequent myocardial remodeling, and heart failure.[1] With an estimated 12.6 million cases globally reported in 2017, AS is the third most common cardiovascular disease in the United States and Europe, with an increasing prevalence of up to 7% in those greater than 65 years of age.[2] The most common etiology is the fibrocalcific thickening of the aortic valve leaflets leading to progressive restricted leaflet

[a] Division of Cardiology, Montefiore Medical Center/Albert Einstein College of Medicine, 111 East 210th street, Bronx, NY 10467, USA; [b] Division of Cardiology, University of Chicago at Northshore University Health System, 1000 Central Street, Evanston, IL 60201, USA; [c] Division of Cardiology, Mount Sinai Morningside. 419 West 114th Street, NY 10025, USA; [d] Division of Cardiology, CEDIMAT. Arturo Logroño, Plaza de la Salud, Dr. Juan Manuel Taveras Rodríguez, C. Pepillo Salcedo esq. Santo Domingo, Dominican Republic; [e] Department of Internal Medicine, University of California Riverside School of Medicine. 900 University Avenue, Riverside, CA 92521, USA; [f] Division of Cardiology, Department of Medicine, Loma Linda University Health, 11234 Anderson Street, Loma Linda, CA 92354, USA
* Corresponding author. Division of Cardiology, Montefiore Medical Center, 111 East 210th street, Bronx, NY 10467.
E-mail address: lslipczukb@montefiore.org

Heart Failure Clin 19 (2023) 491–504
https://doi.org/10.1016/j.hfc.2023.05.010

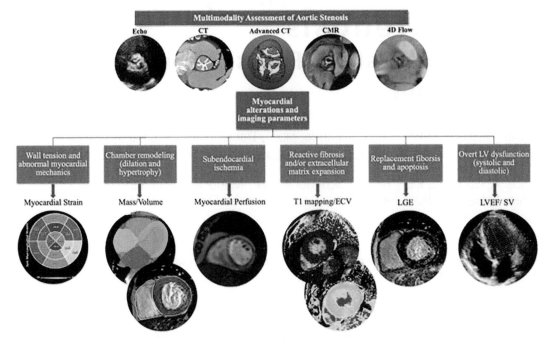

Fig. 1. Multimodality assessment of aortic stenosis: Beyond the valve. CMR, cardiac magnetic resonance; CT, computed tomography; ECV, extracellular volume; LGE, late gadolinium enhancement; LVEF, left ventricular ejection fraction; SV, stroke volume.

opening, with less common etiologies being congenital bicuspid, rheumatic fever, and radiation.[3] It is well-established that severe AS patients who develop symptoms or impaired left ventricular ejection fraction (LVEF) have poor outcomes without aortic valve replacement (AVR).[4] Even though a traditional focus has been on the aortic valve itself, the recent demonstration of subclinical LV remodeling and myocardial fibrosis, together with increased events in patients with traditionally nonsevere AS, has shifted the attention to the myocardium as a complementary marker of the disease process.[5,6] In this review, the authors summarize the available data on the use of multimodality imaging in evaluating the interplay between severe AS and myocardial characterization for risk stratification of patients with AS (**Fig. 1**).

The current 2020 American Heart Association/American College of Cardiology (AHA/ACC) guidelines emphasize a comprehensive assessment of AS and recommend AVR when symptoms or overt myocardial systolic dysfunction (LVEF <50%) ensue. From the initial valve-centered risk stratification, Genereux and colleagues developed an extravalvular staging classification based on cardiac damage. In patients from the PARTNER 2 trial, the stage of cardiac damage by echocardiography was independently associated with increased mortality after AVR (HR 1.46 per each increment in stage, *P*<.0001).[7] Utilization of

multimodality imaging techniques such as echocardiography with global longitudinal strain (GLS), PET, cardiac computed tomography (CT) (**Fig. 2**), and cardiovascular magnetic resonance (CMR) imaging (**Fig. 3**) have provided a wealth of information as to myocardial remodeling secondary to AS. This approach is nevertheless not routinely implemented nor clearly defined in guideline-directed practice for AS, as opposed to regurgitant disease.[4,8]

CHALLENGES OF DISCORDANT ECHOCARDIOGRAPHIC FINDINGS

An accurate assessment of AS severity is crucial for optimal management and timing of AVR. Echocardiography, including Doppler evaluation, is the gold standard imaging modality for grading AS severity, allowing a comprehensive structural and hemodynamic evaluation of the aortic valve and the LV myocardial response, including hypertrophy, remodeling, and ejection fraction. Concordant severe AS is defined in its typical form of high-gradient (HG)-AS as an aortic valve area (AVA) less than 1.0 cm^2 or an indexed AVA (AVAi) less than 0.6 cm^2/m^2 and maximum velocity greater than 4 m/s or a mean gradient greater than 40 mm Hg.[9,10] However, up to 40% of patients present with "discordant grading" on Doppler echocardiography, and it is also referred to as

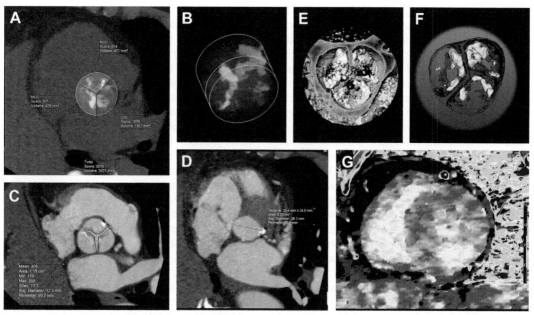

Fig. 2. Comprehensive AS characterization with CCT. (*A, B*) Aortic valve calcium quantification (*TeraRecon*). (*C, D*) AVA and left ventricular outflow tract (LVOT) planimetry. (*E*) VR of the aortic valve. (*F*) Virtual valve biopsy (*Autoplaque*). (*G*) Late iodine enhancement (Z effective image from *Intellispace Portal*).

"low-gradient AS," defined as an AVA consistent with severe (<1.0 cm^2 and <0.6 cm^2/m^2) but with a low gradient/velocity (<40 mm Hg, <4 m/s). In this situation, one must first rule out measurement or calculation errors. Other known sources of error are the poor alignment of the ultrasound beam, the neglect of elevated subvalvular velocities, and the occurrence of pressure recovery.[11]

This discordant pattern may raise uncertainties regarding the true severity of the valve disease

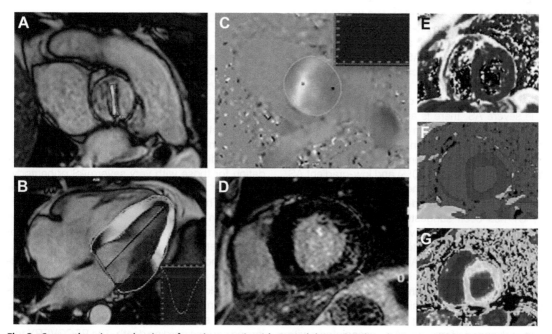

Fig. 3. Comprehensive evaluation of aortic stenosis with CMR. (*A*) Aortic valve planimetry. (*B*) Phase contrast flow and velocity assessment. (*C*) Feature tracking GLS. (*D*) Late gadolinium enhancement. (*E, F*) T2, T1 native, and (*G*) ECV mapping.

and its therapeutic management.[10] The stroke volume index (SVi) is a marker of LV systolic function and an important prognostic factor before and after AVR. Furthermore, because the mean gradient is not only directly related to the stroke volume but also inversely related to the ejection time, a definition of a low-flow state as a mean flow rate less than 200 mL/s has been suggested and associated with a worse prognosis and with a higher likelihood of "pseudo-moderate" gradient and/or pseudo-severe AVA.[12] The discordant low-gradient severe AS entity includes (1) classical low flow (SVi < 35 mL/m^2), low gradient with reduced LVEF (LVEF < 50%); (2) paradoxical low-flow, low-gradient AS with preserved LVEF, seen in patients with small LV cavities (commonly in elderly women with chronic hypertension), severe diastolic dysfunction, atrial fibrillation, significant mitral and tricuspid valvular disease, pulmonary hypertension, right ventricular dysfunction, and cardiac amyloidosis (CA); and (3) normal-flow (SVi > 35 mL/m^2), low-gradient AS, explained by several factors, including a decreased flow rate despite a normal SVi, bradycardia, and/or abnormal arterial hemodynamics (systemic hypertension with prolonged ejection time).[10,12]

In low-flow low-gradient (LF-LG) AS, additional imaging modalities should be considered to confirm AS severity and guide timing to AVR. The use of hybrid imaging for AVA calculation by combining LVOT area by 3D echocardiography or contrast-enhanced CT paired with Doppler velocities has been proposed.[12] The use of CT can lead to overestimation of effective AVA and should be used with caution, and a larger AVA (1.2 cm^2) is considered for severe AS definition. Low-dose Dobutamine stress echocardiography (DSE) may be used to distinguish severe from pseudo-severe in patients with classical LF-LG AS; in true severe AS, there is an increased transaortic velocity and gradient with a fixed valve area after increasing SV greater than 20% with dobutamine. In those patients with inconclusive DSE (defined as failure to increase SV > 20%) and low-gradient AS with preserved LVEF, the aortic valve calcium score (an anatomic, load-independent measure) by CT has been suggested (Class 2a in recent guidelines).[4,12] An aortic valve calcification score greater than 1300 Agatston Units (AU) (420 AU/cm^2) in women or 2000 AU (527 AU/cm^2) in men is considered severe.[13]

The prognostic and clinical significance of the discordant LG-AS remains controversial, with some authors advocating for LG-AS as a severe and advanced form of AS associated with increased interstitial fibrosis, reduced LV longitudinal function, and poor prognosis, whereas others argue for being a less severe phenotype that can be safely monitored clinically. De Azevedo and colleagues, in their analysis of a large cohort (70% conservatively managed patients), confirmed that the survival of discordant LG-AS is better than that of HG-AS and worse than moderate AS patients. At comparable mean gradients, the lower the AVAi, the worse the prognosis, whereas at comparable AVAi, the higher the mean gradient, the worse the prognosis.[9]

Furthermore, in a cohort study including patients with paradoxical LG-AS, moderate AS, and HG-AS, Clavel and colleagues demonstrated that patients with paradoxical LG-AS have a worse prognosis than patients with moderate AS or HG-AS and benefit from AVR.[14] In a population of 1974 patients with moderate AS (AVA >1.0 and ≤ 1.5 cm^2), Stassen and colleagues demonstrated that the discordant patterns are frequent (40%), and LF-LG moderate AS may be associated with increased mortality compared with concordant moderate AS.[15]

Such conflicting data highlight the challenges in predicting future events in severe AS and probably depends on different underlying myocardial phenotypes. Therefore, a more comprehensive approach could guide the appropriate clinical decision-making, integrating symptoms, multiple imaging modalities, and parameters to confirm the actual severity of the valve disease and the extent of myocardial damage caused by AS.

ASYMPTOMATIC SEVERE AORTIC STENOSIS AND THE MYOCARDIUM

Symptoms are often the primary driver for the initial evaluation and/or the reason for referral to cardiology; however, not uncommonly patients with severe AS are asymptomatic at the time of diagnosis.[16] AVR among asymptomatic severe AS patients has a class 1 recommendation for those with LV dysfunction or those undergoing other cardiac surgery and a class 2a recommendation for those with very severe AS or hemodynamic or exercise intolerance with exercise testing.[4] The optimal timing of follow-up and intervention in asymptomatic severe AS remains debated, more so with the exponential growth of transcatheter interventions. A recent systematic review and meta-analysis by Jaiswal and colleagues in asymptomatic severe AS reported that early surgical AVR (n = 765) was safer than conservative management (n = 784) in high-risk AS patients[17] specifically with lower all-cause mortality and sudden cardiac death. The RECOVERY trial randomized 145 patients with very severe asymptomatic AS (AVA 0.75 cm^2, mean gradient ≥50 mm

Hg, peak velocity $\geq$4.5 m/s) and LVEF greater than 50% to an early surgical AVR versus a watchful-waiting strategy.[18] The primary outcome of operative mortality or cardiovascular mortality was significantly lower for early AVR [1% vs 6% (P<.05) at 4 years and 1% vs 26% (P = .003) at 8 years], mostly driven by cardiovascular mortality [1% vs 15% (HR 0.09, 95% CI 0.01–0.67, P<.05)]. Furthermore, in the AVATAR trial, early surgical AVR was compared with conservative therapy in 157 patients with asymptomatic guidelines-defined severe AS.[19] In an intention-to-treat analysis, patients randomized to early surgery had a significantly lower incidence of the primary composite end-point (HR 0.46 [95% CI, 0.23–0.90]; P = .02).

There are currently two ongoing multicenter, randomized controlled clinical trials focusing on outcomes of early AVR in the asymptomatic severe AS population. The EARLY transcatheter aortic valve replacement (TAVR) trial (NCT03042104) intends to investigate outcomes for asymptomatic severe AS patients with high surgical risk who undergo TAVR compared with a watchful waiting strategy. The EVOLVED study (NCT03094143) evaluates the use of biomarkers (high sensitivity (hs)-troponin), electrocardiogram (ECG), and CMR to identify high-risk patients with asymptomatic severe AS and compare outcomes to those patients randomized to receive early AVR versus conservative medical management. These trials could help guide future practice and shape guideline-directed management in this asymptomatic severe AS population.

The outcomes observed from the RECOVERY and AVATAR trial highlight the risk associated with conservative management of asymptomatic severe AS and the need for closer follow-up and frequent reassessment for possible AVR despite LVEF greater than 50%. The use of additional imaging modalities such as CMR and GLS allows better identification of subclinical myocardial dysfunction, dyssynchrony, myocardial injury, and remodeling before the development of overt systolic dysfunction.[9,20]

One meta-analysis by Magne and colleagues investigating the significance of CMR-obtained LV GLS reported that among 1067 patients with asymptomatic severe AS (AVAi < 0.6 cm^2/m^2) and LVEF greater than 50% who did not undergo AVR, a GLS of less than 14.7% was associated with increased all-cause mortality (HR 3.58; 95% CI 1.84–6.99; P<.0001; I^2 = 0, P<.0001).[21] This suggests that compared with LVEF, LV GLS may be a better predictor of survival, thereby serving as a potential tool to guide AVR timing (**Table 1**).

Although impairment of LV GLS in severe AS is load-dependent, it has been associated with increased myocardial fibrosis.[21,22] LV fibrosis can be divided into two types (1) reactive interstitial fibrosis and (2) focal replacement fibrosis. Reactive interstitial fibrosis occurs in the early stages of AS; it can be identified using CMR native T1 mapping or extracellular volume (ECV) fraction derived from native and post-contrast T1 maps (see **Fig. 2**). These two parameters have been validated against histology and correlate with AS severity, LV mass, symptom status, and LV systolic function.[23,24] Moreover, the native T1 value was found to be an independent predictor of outcomes, in addition to other prognosticators such as EuroSCORE II or late gadolinium enhancement (LGE).[25] In 440 patients with severe AS undergoing AVR, Everett and colleagues demonstrated that ECV fraction was the strongest prognostic indicator, even superior to LVEF.[24] Importantly, interstitial fibrosis may be reversible following AVR.[6] On the other hand, replacement fibrosis in the context of AS represents a more advanced stage of the disease. The classic pattern of LGE uptake has been described as intramyocardial or "mid-wall." In a large study involving 674 patients with severe AS undergoing AVR, the presence and amount of LGE was a strong independent predictor of worse outcomes (every 1% increase in LGE mortality hazard ratio increased by 11% and cardiovascular mortality by 8%).[26]

Focusing on the left atrium (LA), Tan and colleagues sought to investigate the prognostic performance of LA strain in relation to clinical, echocardiographic variables and N-terminal-pro brain natriuretic peptide (NT-proBNP) in 173 patients with asymptomatic or minimally symptomatic severe AS with LVEF greater than 50%.[27] They found that LA strain parameters outperformed other key echocardiographic variables and NT-ProBNP in predicting clinical outcomes. In addition, in a similar asymptomatic severe AS cohort of 248 patients with LVEF$\geq$50%, LA strain rate and AVA correlated to the presence of HF with preserved EF.[28]

The above-mentioned data show the extensive recent progress in the subclinical impact of severe AS and the role of several biomarkers that allow early recognition of those high-risk patients who may benefit from prompt intervention.

EFFECTS OF MODERATE AORTIC STENOSIS ON THE MYOCARDIUM

Current guidelines do not recommend AVR for isolated moderate AS unless cardiac surgery is considered for another indication.[4] Nonetheless,

Table 1
Advanced myocardial imaging biomarkers in aortic stenosis

Echocardiography	CMR[5,6,24,53,54]	CCT
LV GLS[21,55] • Abnormal even when EF $\geq$ 50% • Strong prognostic value • > −14.7% was associated with a 2.5-fold increased risk of death LV myocardial work[56] • Myocardial deformation + LV afterload • Associated with heart failure incidence	LGE • Present in 27%–51% • Associated with AS severity, LV systolic, and diastolic dysfunction • Predicts mortality. • Pattern: Subendocardial (ischemic) vs Mid-myocardial (nonischemic) • Replacement fibrosis (irreversible) Native T1 • Diffuse fibrosis • Correlated with collagen volume fraction • Increased with disease severity ECV CMR • ECV > 28% in up to 54% with severe AS • Predicts mortality • Interstitial fibrosis (reversible with AVR) T2 (edema/inflammation) FT-GLS • Associated with outcomes post-AVR Stress perfusion • Coronary epicardial disease • Microvascular ischemia	ECV$_{CT}$[57] • Correlated with ECV$_{CMR}$ and histology • Prognostic value in AS + TTR-amyloid pre-TAVR

Abbreviations: CCT, cardiovascular computed tomography; CMR, cardiovascular magnetic resonance; ECV, extracellular volume; FT, feature tracking; GLS, global longitudinal strain; LGE, late gadolinium enhancement; LV, left ventricle; TAVR, transcatheter aortic valve replacement; TTR, transthyretin.

the severity of AS and LV systolic function are continuous variables, and structural repercussions in the LV myocardium can occur in parallel with a progressive increase in AS severity. In patients with HF with reduced ejection fraction (HFrEF), the simultaneous presence of moderate AS may further hamper LV systolic function by increasing afterload. In a recent meta-analysis, by Coisne and colleagues,[29] among a total of 25 studies (12,143 moderate AS patients, 3.7 years of follow-up), pooled rates per 100 person-years were 9.0 (95% CI: 6.9–11.7) for all-cause death. The investigators depicted that moderate AS seems to be associated with a mortality risk higher than no or mild AS but lower than severe AS, which increases in specific population subsets.

Before reaching the stage of overt LV dysfunction, through the use of CMR, several studies have demonstrated the presence and prognostic implications of nonischemic myocardial fibrosis

in patients with moderate or severe AS.[30] In 143 patients with moderate (40%) and severe AS, Dweck and colleagues showed that 38% had mid-wall LGE uptake patterns and was an independent predictor of mortality regardless of the presence of concomitant ischemic subendocardial scar.[26] Interestingly, in that study, more than one-half of the patients with mid-wall fibrosis who died had only moderate AS, and they would not have been considered for AVR under standard-of-care practice.

It has been shown that an LVEF $\geq$50% often already represents subclinical myocardial dysfunction and a value < 60% in the presence of moderate AS could be considered abnormal.[31] In moderate AS, LV GLS may have an additional value in assessing early myocardial dysfunction. In 287 patients with moderate AS and LVEF $\geq$50%, Zhu and colleagues showed that patients with more impaired LV GLS (>−15.2%) had higher mortality rates ($P < .001$).[32] These findings were consistent among patients with LVEF $\geq$60% and those who underwent AVR. Moreover, Stassen and colleagues found that patients with moderate AS and preserved LVEF, but impaired LV GLS (>−16%) had equally worse outcomes than patients with reduced LVEF.[33] Similarly to severe AS, the concept of "cardiac damage" has been evaluated recently in 1245 patients with moderate AS and significantly higher mortality was found with increasing extent of abnormalities.[34]

Along with imaging parameters of LV remodeling, specific myocardial biomarkers may alert of an ongoing maladaptive response to pressure overload. For example, in 261 patients with moderate AS, higher levels of NT-proBNP were associated with increased mortality rates, even after adjusting for age, gender, comorbidities, and echocardiographic LV parameters.[35]

Evidence continues to accumulate (**Table 2**), supporting the notion of AS severity as a continuous variable, with increasing AS severity imposing an increased pressure load on the LV. Ongoing randomized trials may likely answer whether an earlier AVR may improve outcomes in selected patients with moderate AS. The TAVR UNLOAD trial (NCT02661451) aims to investigate the effect of mechanical unloading with TAVR in patients with symptomatic moderate AS and LVEF less than 50%. The PROGRESS trial (NCT04889872) will include patients $\geq$65 year old and moderate AS with cardiac dysfunction or symptoms to evaluate the benefit of optimal medical therapy (OMT) plus transfemoral TAVR versus OMT alone. Finally, the EXPAND II trial (NCT05149755) will compare OMT with TAVR in patients with symptomatic moderate AS and one of the following: one heart failure decompensation episode in the past year, elevated NT-proBNP levels, reduced GLS or E/e' over 14.

AORTIC STENOSIS AND CARDIAC AMYLOIDOSIS

CA is characterized by an extracellular deposit of amyloid fibrils within the myocardium and other cardiac structures; it shares several common features with AS, with a worse prognosis.[36] Overall, transthyretin (TTR) is the most prevalent type of CA associated with AS, especially in men aged greater than 70 years.[37] LV myocardial infiltration by amyloid fibrils causes increased biventricular wall thickness and stiffness, impairing LV diastolic and longitudinal systolic function and leading to restrictive cardiomyopathy.[38] Diastolic HF with preserved LVEF is the most common presentation, but nearly one-third of patients may have HFrEF.[39]

These features are also common in patients with severe AS, which may mask the presence of a concomitant CA. In addition, aortic valve infiltration by amyloid may contribute to the initiation and progression of AS.[40] Limited data are available on CA prevalence either isolated or associated with AS. A recent study discovered CA in 11.8% of AS patients through bone scintigraphy and exclusion of light chain (AL)-CA.[41]

Until now, there has been no recommendation or consensus on whether patients with AS should be systematically screened for CA. The TTR-CA screening and diagnosis protocol is similar in AS and the general population, but it is more challenging because AS and CA share several features. In patients with AS, which raise "Red Flags" for suspicion of CA, it should be tested. TTE features such as a mitral annulus S' velocity $\leq$6 cm/s are useful in screening for CA in patients with AS and preserved LVEF.[42] LV GLS is often markedly reduced and preserved at the apex in CA, but the apical sparing may also be observed in patients with AS and no CA.[43] A paradoxical (preserved LVEF) LF-LG AS pattern should also raise suspicion for CA.[42]

The high prevalence of low-flow state in patients with CA may be explained by severe concentric LV and LA remodeling, impairment of diastolic filling, markedly reduced LV longitudinal systolic function, and RV remodeling and dysfunction.[44] In patients with CA, DSE often fails to increase LV outflow significantly and thus provides inconclusive results. Hence, quantifying AV calcium burden using non-contrast CT appears to be the most appropriate imaging modality to confirm AS severity in patients with CA.[45]

Diagnostic features by CMR (**Table 3**) offer the possibility of differentiating CA from other cardiomyopathies associated with LV hypertrophy. Still, 15% of CMR examinations may be normal in patients with CA.[38] In the past decade, CT has gained attention as a potential tool to assess ECV, a marker of myocardial fibrosis that increases moderately with diffuse fibrosis but massively with CA. Kidoh and colleagues[46] described the sensitivity of ECV for detecting CA in CT TAVR as 90% and a specificity of 92% (**Fig. 4**). ECV CT can reliably detect dual AS-amyloid pathology with only 3 min on top of the standard CT imaging evaluation and a small radiation burden ($\sim$2.3 mSv).[46] The measured ECV CT does not just help detect but to track the degree of infiltration. Commonly used in the pre-TAVR evaluation, cardiac CT offers a possible one-stop-shop analysis of valvular morphology, AS severity, cardiac function, and myocardial characterization. Recently, CT-GLS was demonstrated feasible to

Table 2
Summary of literature involving moderate aortic stenosis

Study	Type	Population	Female sex	Moderate as	Follow-up	Primary Endpoint	Results
Van Gils et al,[58] 2017	Retrospective multicenter	305 patients with moderate AS and LVEF<50%	25%	305	4 y	All-cause death, AVR, and HFH	• Primary endpoint in 61% • Male sex, NYHA III/IV, and Vmax were independent predictors
Strange et al,[59] 2019	Registry: National Echocardiographic Database of Australia (NEDA)	241,303 individuals with full spectrum of AS.	37% (of mod AS patients)	3315	5 y	All-cause death and CV mortality	• Primary end point in 56% of moderate AS and 67% in severe AS • Markedly increased risk (adjusted for age, sex, LVEF, and so forth) with AV mean gradient ≧20 mm Hg or Vmax≧3 m/s
Dweck et al,[26] 2011	Prospective registry	143 patients with CMR	33%	57(40%)	2 y	All-cause mortality	• Mid-wall fibrosis/LGE is an independent predictor of the primary endpoint (HR: 5.35; 95% CI: 1.16–24.56) • 50% of patients with mid-wall LGE had moderate AS • 50% of mid-wall LGE patients who died had moderate AS
Zhu et al,[32] 2020	Retrospective	287 patients with moderate AS and LVEF≥ 50%.	53%	287	3.9 y	All-cause mortality	• Primary end point in 36% • GLS > −15.2% had higher mortality (HR 2.62 [95% CI 1.69–4.06]), even in those with LVEF≥60% and those undergoing AVR
Stassen et al,[60] 2022	Muti-registry data	1931 patients	48%	1931	3 y	All-cause mortality	• Concentric LVH in 36%. • LVH independently associated with mortality (HR 1.25 [95% CI 1.01–1.55])

| Ito et al,[35] 2020 | Retrospective | 261 patients with moderate AS | 36% | 261 | 2.7 y | All-cause mortality | • Primary end point in 52%
 • NT-proBNP >888 pg/dL had higher mortality
 • Higher NT-pro BNP associated with higher mortality rate (HR 3.11 [95% CI 1.78–5.46]), even in those undergoing AVR |

Abbreviations: AS, aortic stenosis; AVR, aortic valve replacement; CI, confidence interval; GLS, global longitudinal strain; HFH, heart failure hospitalization; HR, hazard ratio; LGE, late gadolinium enhancement; LVEF, left ventricular ejection fraction; LVH, left ventricular hypertrophy; NT-proBNP, N-terminal-pro brain natriuretic peptide; NYHA, New York Heart Association.

Table 3
Red flags imaging criteria to suspect and confirm cardiac amyloidosis in patients with aortic stenosis

Demographics	Elderly ≥ 65 y, Male Sex, African Descendant
Clinical features	HFpEF, RV failure (ascites, edema), disproportionate HF symptoms, conduction abnormalities, unilateral/bilateral carpal tunnel syndrome, deafness, lumbar spinal stenosis
Biomarkers	Chronic troponin ↑ without significant coronary artery disease (CAD)/chronic kidney disease (CKD), NT-proBNP/BNP ↑ disproportionate to AS severity in the absence of renal failure
ECG	Discordant low-voltage and LV wall thickness, pseudo-infarction pattern (Q waves) without history of myocardial infarction
Echocardiography	LV wall thickening (≥15 mm) disproportionate to AS severity Myocardial granular sparkling Severe LV concentric remodeling (RWT >0.5) Severity of LV diastolic dysfunction (Grade ≥2; E/e'>15) disproportionate to LVH Severe LV longitudinal systolic dysfunction with apical sparing LV global longitudinal strain ≥ −12% and/or apex/basal longitudinal strain ratio >2 Moderate/severe pulmonary hypertension Mitral S' ≤6 cm/s RV wall hypertrophy (≥5 mm) Biatrial dilatation Atrial septal thickening Atrioventricular valve thickening (>2 mm)
CMR	Elevated native T1 mapping and extracellular volume Abnormal gadolinium kinetics with short T1 inversion scout sequences Circumferential and extensive late gadolinium enhancement (subendocardial, basal predominance)
Diagnostic confirmation	Serum/urine monoclonal free light chain protein (for AL-CA) Additional tissue biopsy offten required Bone scintigraphy (for TTR-CA). Histology on endomyocardial and/or extracardiac biopsies.

Abbreviations: AS, aortic stenosis; BNP, brain natriuretic peptide; CA, cardiac amyloidosis; CMR, cardiac magnetic resonance; ECG, electrocardiogram; HFpEF, heart failure with preserved ejection fraction; LV, left ventricular; NT-proBNP, N-terminal pro-brain natriuretic peptide; TTR-CA, transthyretin cardiac amyloidosis.

detect subclinical myocardial changes in AS with a moderate correlation between CT-GLS and TTE (r = 0.62, P<.001).[47]

The clinical impact of myocardial amyloid deposition in patients with AS remains unclear. Further studies are needed to determine the optimal approaches for the screening and treatment of CA in patients with AS. Finally, specific guidelines should be developed to guide the heart team in deciding the type and the timing of treatment in symptomatic patients with severe AS and concomitant CA.

UTILIZATION OF FLUORODEOXYGLUCOSE PET IN EVALUATION OF AORTIC STENOSIS

Fluoro-2-deoxyglucose PET (FDG-PET) imaging can provide metabolic and functional assessment in evaluating AS and its effect on the myocardium. An increased glycolytic metabolic activity represents aortic valve inflammatory cell activity. Dweck and colleagues[48] demonstrated increased 18F-FDG uptake in hypermetabolic or inflamed tissues, and 18F-sodium fluoride (NaF) activity (a marker for active calcification) was noted to be greater than FDG activity in advanced AS.[49] Understanding that AS is an active local inflammatory condition not limited to the aortic valve, PET can provide an alternative method to evaluate the disease progression, risk stratification, and guide therapy in patients with AS.

In addition, as demonstrated by Zhou and colleagues, myocardial evaluation is also possible. Their work indicated that myocardial flow reserve (MFR) and stress myocardial blood flow were associated with adverse LV characteristics,

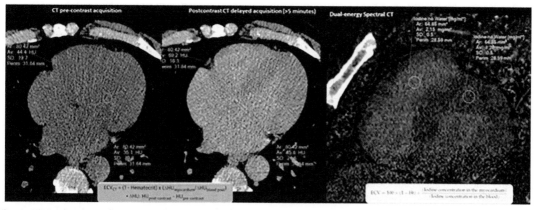

Fig. 4. CT evaluation of myocardial extracellular volume with conventional single energy scanner. Measurements were performed with *Philips Intellispace Portal v12.0.* CT evaluation of myocardial extracellular volume using dual-layer Spectral CT. Only one acquisition is required (delayed >5 minutes post-contrast) to obtain the iodine concentration of myocardium and blood poll. Images were acquired using *Philips IQon 64* scanner and analyzed with Philips Intellispace Portal v12.0.

myocardial injury, and increased wall stress in AS.[50] MFR improved after AVR, suggesting that it may be an early marker for myocardial decompensation, likely due to the increased pressure gradient and wall stress leading to subendocardial ischemia and compounded by inherent microvascular dysfunction from common comorbidities, such as hypertension, CAD, and diabetes. Furthermore, PET could help differentiate between mimickers of LV remodeling secondary to AS, especially through the hybrid PET-MR approach that would allow characterization of LV volumes, mass, EF, and LGE burden.[51]

FUTURE PERSPECTIVES

Cardiac damage staging by echocardiography can predict both post-AVR outcomes and reverse remodeling beyond valve characteristics.[52] Although the valve is the primary insult, its interplay with the left ventricular myocardial response can manifest maladaptive changes earlier and ultimately determine the patient's prognosis and adaptive capabilities. Consequently, decisions regarding intervention, including timing and patient selection, should contemplate the myocardial response. New multimodality imaging tools, such as strain, parametric mapping, and LGE, present further opportunities to provide cardiac staging as a continuum. Of particular interest is the ability to identify the critical transition from adaptive, potentially reversible myocardial remodeling to maladaptive and potentially irreversible remodeling. Advanced imaging tools have unique capabilities to predict adverse myocardial remodeling and therefore refine timing for intervention in these patients, but they are still largely under-utilized, likely

due to limited availability, standardization, and prospective validation. New trials are needed to investigate whether an imaging-guided earlier AVR approach may improve outcomes in patients with severe and moderate AS.

CLINICS CARE POINTS

- Accurate assessment of aortic stenosis severity is crucial for optimal management and timing of aortic valve replacement (AVR).
- Cardiac damage staging by echocardiography can predict both post-AVR outcomes and reverse remodeling beyond valve characteristics.
- New multimodality imaging tools, such as strain, parametric mapping, and LGE, present further opportunities to provide cardiac staging as a continuum.

DISCLOSURE

P Pina and D Lorenzatti are supported by grants from Amgen, United States and Philips, Netherlands. L Slipczuk has received an honorarium from Amgen, BMS, and Philips and grant support from Amgen and Philips. P Parwani is a consultant for Medtronic and Astrazeneca.

REFERENCES

1. Boskovski MT, Gleason TG. Current Therapeutic Options in Aortic Stenosis. Circ Res 2021;128(9): 1398–417.

2. Choi YJ, Son JW, Kim EK, et al. Epidemiologic Profile of Patients With Valvular Heart Disease in Korea: A Nationwide Hospital-Based Registry Study. J Cardiovasc Imaging 2023;31(1):51–61.

3. Yadgir S, Johnson CO, Aboyans V, et al. Global, Regional, and National Burden of Calcific Aortic Valve and Degenerative Mitral Valve Diseases, 1990-2017. Circulation 2020;141(21):1670–80.

4. Otto CM, Nishimura RA, Bonow RO, et al. 2020 ACC/AHA Guideline for the Management of Patients With Valvular Heart Disease: Executive Summary: A Report of the American College of Cardiology/American Heart Association Joint Committee on Clinical Practice Guidelines. Circulation 2021;143(5):e35–71.

5. Ajmone Marsan N, Delgado V, Shah DJ, et al. Valvular heart disease: shifting the focus to the myocardium. Eur Heart J 2023;44(1):28–40.

6. Treibel TA, Kozor R, Schofield R, et al. Reverse Myocardial Remodeling Following Valve Replacement in Patients With Aortic Stenosis. J Am Coll Cardiol 2018;71(8):860–71.

7. Généreux P, Pibarot P, Redfors B, et al. Staging classification of aortic stenosis based on the extent of cardiac damage. Eur Heart J 2017;38(45):3351–8.

8. Bing R, Cavalcante JL, Everett RJ, et al. Imaging and Impact of Myocardial Fibrosis in Aortic Stenosis. JACC Cardiovasc Imaging 2019;12(2):283–96.

9. De Azevedo D, Tribouilloy C, Maréchaux S, et al. Prognostic Implications of Discordant Low-Gradient Severe Aortic Stenosis: Comprehensive Analysis of a Large Multicenter Registry. JACC Adv 2023;2(2):100254.

10. Guzzetti E, Annabi MS, Pibarot P, et al. Multimodality Imaging for Discordant Low-Gradient Aortic Stenosis: Assessing the Valve and the Myocardium. Front Cardiovasc Med 2020;7. Available at: https://www.frontiersin.org/articles/10.3389/fcvm.2020.570689. Accessed May 9, 2023.

11. Niederberger J, Schima H, Maurer G, et al. Importance of Pressure Recovery for the Assessment of Aortic Stenosis by Doppler Ultrasound. Circulation 1996;94(8):1934–40.

12. Delgado V, Clavel MA, Hahn RT, et al. How Do We Reconcile Echocardiography, Computed Tomography, and Hybrid Imaging in Assessing Discordant Grading of Aortic Stenosis Severity? JACC Cardiovasc Imaging 2019;12(2):267–82.

13. Pawade T, Sheth T, Guzzetti E, et al. Why and How to Measure Aortic Valve Calcification in Patients With Aortic Stenosis. JACC Cardiovasc Imaging 2019;12(9):1835–48.

14. Clavel MA, Dumesnil JG, Capoulade R, et al. Outcome of patients with aortic stenosis, small valve area, and low-flow, low-gradient despite preserved left ventricular ejection fraction. J Am Coll Cardiol 2012;60(14):1259–67.

15. Stassen J, Ewe SH, Singh GK, et al. Prevalence and Prognostic Implications of Discordant Grading and Flow-Gradient Patterns in Moderate Aortic Stenosis. J Am Coll Cardiol 2022;80(7):666–76.

16. Lindman BR, Clavel MA, Mathieu P, et al. Calcific aortic stenosis. Nat Rev Dis Primer 2016;2:16006.

17. Jaiswal V, Khan N, Jaiswal A, et al. Early surgery vs conservative management among asymptomatic aortic stenosis: A systematic review and meta-analysis. Int J Cardiol Heart Vasc 2022;43:101125.

18. Kang DH, Park SJ, Lee SA, et al. Early Surgery or Conservative Care for Asymptomatic Aortic Stenosis. N Engl J Med 2020;382(2):111–9.

19. Banovic M, Putnik S, Penicka M, et al. Aortic Valve Replacement Versus Conservative Treatment in Asymptomatic Severe Aortic Stenosis: The AVATAR Trial. Circulation 2022;145(9):648–58.

20. Lancellotti P, Donal E, Magne J, et al. Impact of global left ventricular afterload on left ventricular function in asymptomatic severe aortic stenosis: a two-dimensional speckle-tracking study. Eur J Echocardiogr J Work Group Echocardiogr Eur Soc Cardiol 2010;11(6):537–43.

21. Magne J, Cosyns B, Popescu BA, et al. Distribution and Prognostic Significance of Left Ventricular Global Longitudinal Strain in Asymptomatic Significant Aortic Stenosis: An Individual Participant Data Meta-Analysis. JACC Cardiovasc Imaging 2019;12(1):84–92.

22. Kostakou PM, Tryfou ES, Kostopoulos VS, et al. Segmentally impaired left ventricular longitudinal strain: a new predictive diagnostic parameter for asymptomatic patients with severe aortic stenosis and preserved ejection fraction. Perfusion 2022;37(4):402–9.

23. Chin CWL, Everett RJ, Kwiecinski J, et al. Myocardial Fibrosis and Cardiac Decompensation in Aortic Stenosis. JACC Cardiovasc Imaging 2017;10(11):1320–33.

24. Everett RJ, Treibel TA, Fukui M, et al. Extracellular Myocardial Volume in Patients With Aortic Stenosis. J Am Coll Cardiol 2020;75(3):304–16.

25. Lee JM, Choi KH, Koo BK, et al. Prognostic Implications of Plaque Characteristics and Stenosis Severity in Patients With Coronary Artery Disease. J Am Coll Cardiol 2019;73(19):2413–24.

26. Dweck MR, Joshi S, Murigu T, et al. Midwall fibrosis is an independent predictor of mortality in patients with aortic stenosis. J Am Coll Cardiol 2011;58(12):1271–9.

27. Tan ESJ, Jin X, Oon YY, et al. Prognostic Value of Left Atrial Strain in Aortic Stenosis: A Competing Risk Analysis. J Am Soc Echocardiogr Off Publ Am Soc Echocardiogr 2023;36(1):29–37.e5.

28. Mateescu AD, Călin A, Beladan CC, et al. Left Atrial Dysfunction as an Independent Correlate of Heart Failure Symptoms in Patients With Severe Aortic

Stenosis and Preserved Left Ventricular Ejection Fraction. J Am Soc Echocardiogr Off Publ Am Soc Echocardiogr 2019;32(2):257–66.

29. Coisne A, Scotti A, Latib A, et al. Impact of Moderate Aortic Stenosis on Long-Term Clinical Outcomes. JACC Cardiovasc Interv 2022;15(16):1664–74.

30. Stassen J, Ewe SH, Pio SM, et al. Managing Patients With Moderate Aortic Stenosis. JACC Cardiovasc Imaging 2023. https://doi.org/10.1016/j.jcmg.2022.12.013.

31. Ito S, Miranda WR, Nkomo VT, et al. Reduced Left Ventricular Ejection Fraction in Patients With Aortic Stenosis. J Am Coll Cardiol 2018;71(12):1313–21.

32. Zhu D, Ito S, Miranda WR, et al. Left Ventricular Global Longitudinal Strain Is Associated With Long-Term Outcomes in Moderate Aortic Stenosis. Circ Cardiovasc Imaging 2020;13(4):e009958.

33. Stassen J, Pio SM, Ewe SH, et al. Left Ventricular Global Longitudinal Strain in Patients with Moderate Aortic Stenosis. J Am Soc Echocardiogr Off Publ Am Soc Echocardiogr 2022;35(8):791–800.e4.

34. Amanullah MR, Pio SM, Ng ACT, et al. Prognostic Implications of Associated Cardiac Abnormalities Detected on Echocardiography in Patients With Moderate Aortic Stenosis. JACC Cardiovasc Imaging 2021;14(9):1724–37.

35. Ito S, Miranda WR, Jaffe AS, et al. Prognostic Value of N-Terminal Pro-form B-Type Natriuretic Peptide in Patients With Moderate Aortic Stenosis. Am J Cardiol 2020;125(10):1566–70.

36. d'Humières T, Fard D, Damy T, et al. Outcome of patients with cardiac amyloidosis admitted to an intensive care unit for acute heart failure. Arch Cardiovasc Dis 2018;111(10):582–90.

37. Ruberg FL, Grogan M, Hanna M, et al. Transthyretin Amyloid Cardiomyopathy: JACC State-of-the-Art Review. J Am Coll Cardiol 2019;73(22):2872–91.

38. Ternacle J, Krapf L, Mohty D, et al. Aortic Stenosis and Cardiac Amyloidosis: JACC Review Topic of the Week. J Am Coll Cardiol 2019;74(21):2638–51.

39. González-López E, Gallego-Delgado M, Guzzo-Merello G, et al. Wild-type transthyretin amyloidosis as a cause of heart failure with preserved ejection fraction. Eur Heart J 2015;36(38):2585–94.

40. Audet A, Côté N, Couture C, et al. Amyloid substance within stenotic aortic valves promotes mineralization. Histopathology 2012;61(4):610–9.

41. Nitsche C, Scully PR, Patel KP, et al. Prevalence and Outcomes of Concomitant Aortic Stenosis and Cardiac Amyloidosis. J Am Coll Cardiol 2021;77(2):128–39.

42. Castaño A, Narotsky DL, Hamid N, et al. Unveiling transthyretin cardiac amyloidosis and its predictors among elderly patients with severe aortic stenosis undergoing transcatheter aortic valve replacement. Eur Heart J 2017;38(38):2879–87.

43. Abecasis J, Lopes P, Santos RR, et al. Prevalence and significance of relative apical sparing in aortic stenosis: insights from an echo and cardiovascular magnetic resonance study of patients referred for surgical aortic valve replacement. Eur Heart J - Cardiovasc Imaging 2023. https://doi.org/10.1093/ehjci/jead032. jead032.

44. Galat A, Guellich A, Bodez D, et al. Aortic stenosis and transthyretin cardiac amyloidosis: the chicken or the egg? Eur Heart J 2016;37(47):3525–31.

45. Treibel TA, Fontana M, Gilbertson JA, et al. Occult Transthyretin Cardiac Amyloid in Severe Calcific Aortic Stenosis: Prevalence and Prognosis in Patients Undergoing Surgical Aortic Valve Replacement. Circ Cardiovasc Imaging 2016;9(8):e005066.

46. Kidoh M, Oda S, Takashio S, et al. CT Extracellular Volume Fraction versus Myocardium-to-Lumen Signal Ratio for Cardiac Amyloidosis. Radiology 2022. https://doi.org/10.1148/radiol.220542.

47. Fukui M, Xu J, Abdelkarim I, et al. Global longitudinal strain assessment by computed tomography in severe aortic stenosis patients - Feasibility using feature tracking analysis. J Cardiovasc Comput Tomogr 2019;13(2):157–62.

48. Dweck MR, Jones C, Joshi NV, et al. Assessment of valvular calcification and inflammation by positron emission tomography in patients with aortic stenosis. Circulation 2012;125(1):76–86.

49. Marincheva-Savcheva G, Subramanian S, Qadir S, et al. Imaging of the aortic valve using fluorodeoxyglucose positron emission tomography increased valvular fluorodeoxyglucose uptake in aortic stenosis. J Am Coll Cardiol 2011;57(25):2507–15.

50. Zhou W, Sun YP, Divakaran S, et al. Association of Myocardial Blood Flow Reserve With Adverse Left Ventricular Remodeling in Patients With Aortic Stenosis: The Microvascular Disease in Aortic Stenosis (MIDAS) Study. JAMA Cardiol 2022;7(1):93–9.

51. Nordström J, Kvernby S, Kero T, et al. Left-ventricular volumes and ejection fraction from cardiac ECG-gated 15O-water positron emission tomography compared to cardiac magnetic resonance imaging using simultaneous hybrid PET/MR. J Nucl Cardiol 2022. https://doi.org/10.1007/s12350-022-03154-7.

52. Parikh PB. Predicting Futility in Aortic Stenosis: What's the Holdup? J Am Coll Cardiol 2022;80(8):801–3.

53. Lee SP, Lee W, Lee JM, et al. Assessment of diffuse myocardial fibrosis by using MR imaging in asymptomatic patients with aortic stenosis. Radiology 2015;274(2):359–69.

54. Fukui M, Annabi MS, Rosa VEE, et al. Comprehensive myocardial characterization using cardiac magnetic resonance associates with outcomes in low gradient severe aortic stenosis. Eur Heart J Cardiovasc Imaging 2022;24(1):46–58.

55. Thellier N, Altes A, Appert L, et al. Prognostic Importance of Left Ventricular Global Longitudinal Strain in Patients with Severe Aortic Stenosis and

Preserved Ejection Fraction. J Am Soc Echocardiogr Off Publ Am Soc Echocardiogr 2020;33(12):1454–64.

56. Fortuni F, Butcher SC, van der Kley F, et al. Left Ventricular Myocardial Work in Patients with Severe Aortic Stenosis. J Am Soc Echocardiogr Off Publ Am Soc Echocardiogr 2021;34(3):257–66.

57. Treibel TA, Patel KP, Cavalcante JL. Extracellular Volume Imaging in Aortic Stenosis During Routine Pre-TAVR Cardiac Computed Tomography. JACC Cardiovasc Imaging 2020;13(12):2602–4.

58. van Gils L, Clavel MA, Vollema EM, et al. Prognostic Implications of Moderate Aortic Stenosis in Patients With Left Ventricular Systolic Dysfunction. J Am Coll Cardiol 2017;69(19):2383–92.

59. Strange G, Stewart S, Celermajer D, et al. Poor Long-Term Survival in Patients With Moderate Aortic Stenosis. J Am Coll Cardiol 2019;74(15):1851–63.

60. Stassen J, Ewe SH, Hirasawa K, et al. Left ventricular remodelling patterns in patients with moderate aortic stenosis. Eur Heart J Cardiovasc Imaging 2022;23(10):1326–35.

Tricuspid Regurgitation and Right Heart Failure
The Role of Imaging in Defining Pathophysiology, Presentation, and Novel Management Strategies

Vratika Agarwal, MD*, Rebecca Hahn, MD

KEYWORDS

- Tricuspid regurgitation • Right heart failure • Transcatheter tricuspid valve intervention

KEY POINTS

- Understanding the anatomy of tricuspid valve and physiology of tricuspid valve function, is integral to understanding the development of tricuspid regurgitation and the relationhip to right heart and pulmonary vascular function.
- Multimodality imaging plays a crucial role in delineating the etiology of TR, anatomy of the tricuspid valve as well as effects of TR on pulmonary vascular system and right ventricle.
- Defining the morphology and clinical etiology of TR and understanding the associated differences in outcome is paramount to both the optimization of current treatments as well as for development of new treatment options for TR.

During the last few years, there has been a substantial shift in efforts to understand and manage secondary or functional tricuspid regurgitation (TR) given its prevalence, adverse prognostic impact, and symptom burden associated with progressive right heart failure.[1] The previously "forgotten valve" has gained tremendous attention due to advances in novel treatment strategies; however, the timing and impact of intervention is not well understood. Recent study shows that the age-adjusted prevalence of TR is about 0.55% with an increasing incidence in population aged older than 75 years[2] with secondary or functional TR the most common cause.[3] Understanding the pathophysiology of TR and right heart failure is crucial for determining the best treatment strategy and improving outcomes. In this article, we review the complex relationship between right heart structural and hemodynamic changes that drive the pathophysiology of secondary TR and discuss the role of multimodality imaging in the diagnosis, management, and determination of outcomes.

TRICUSPID VALVE AND RIGHT HEART ANATOMY

To understand the pathophysiologic relationship between right heart structure and function and mechanisms of secondary TR, it is important to appreciate the complex anatomy of the tricuspid valve (TV) and the right ventricle (RV). TV is distinct from the other valves in its anatomical variability and complexity. The TV apparatus is composed of (1) the tricuspid anulus (TA), (2) leaflets, (3) subvalvular chordae, and (4) papillary muscles.[4] The TV is the largest valve in the body, with a saddle-shaped TA (high points at the septum and lateral wall) with a dynamic change in shape during the

Division of Cardiology, Department of Medicine, Columbia University Medical Center/ New York Presbyterian Hospital, 177 Fort Washington Avenue, Room 5C-501, New York, NY 10032, USA
* Corresponding author. 177 Fort Washington Avenue, Room 5C-501, New York, NY 10032.
E-mail address: va2374@cumc.columbia.edu

Heart Failure Clin 19 (2023) 505–523
https://doi.org/10.1016/j.hfc.2023.03.008
1551-7136/23/© 2023 Elsevier Inc. All rights reserved.

cardiac cycle to ensure maximum flow across the valve in diastole and achieve coaptation during systole.[5] There is very little fibrous tissue or collagen along the RV free wall segment of the TA[6] with greater cellularity and organized elastic fibers in men compared with women.[7] Normal women also have larger indexed TA dimensions and area and thus may be predisposed to developing TR. In fact, by the eighth decade of life, significant TR is 4 times more prevalent in women than in men.[8] Atrial fibrillation results in dilatation of the TA and blunting of the dynamic change in TA shape, contributing to the progression of TR.[9]

The tricuspid leaflets are thin and highly variable in size and number.[10] The main support for the anterior and posterior leaflets is complex chordal arcades that originate from a large anterior papillary muscle, attached to the moderator band and lateral RV wall. A variable number of posterior papillary muscles subtend the variable number of posterior leaflets. Unique to this right atrioventricular valve are the numerous direct chordal attachments from the interventricular septum to the septal leaflet(s) and often portions of the anterior leaflet. Alteration of any of these structures may lead to malcoaptation the leaflet tips and TR.

The RV is the anterior most chamber of the heart and lies close to the chest wall and can be divided into 3 parts—the inlet, the body, and the outlet.[11,12] Muscle fibers are arranged in 2 layers with the outer myocytes arranged circumferentially and inner layer of longitudinal fibers. The RV contracts by 3 separate mechanisms[1]: movement of the free wall toward the septum, which produces a bellowing effect[2]; traction on the free wall at the points of attachment to left ventricular (LV) as well as contraction of the superficial fibres connecting the LV-RV; and contraction of the longitudinal fibers, which shortens the long axis and draws the TA toward the apex.[11] Unlike the LV, which relies on oblique muscle fibers, the majority of the RV function is driven by contraction of the longitudinal muscle fibers. However, RV systolic function is highly reliant on pulmonary pressures (afterload), preload as well as contractile function of the RV. The RV has long been thought to be more sensitive than the LV to acute increases in afterload[13] with experimental models showing that a pressure load on the RV is less well tolerated than a volume load.[14] In response to pressure overload, the RV remodeling is initially adaptive, characterized by more concentric hypertrophy with mild RV dilatation, with preserved systolic and diastolic function.[15] With progression of the primary disease process, there is maladaptive remodeling associated with more eccentric hypertrophy and thus marked RV dilatation and reduced systolic and diastolic function.[16] With RV dilatation, there is a loss of longitudinal RV function; however, recruitment of circumferential myocytes preserves RV stroke volume.

PATHOPHYSIOLOGY OF SECONDARY TRICUSPID REGURGITATION

Several studies evaluating predictors of TR severity and progression have resulted in a more comprehensive understanding of TR pathophysiology. Maladaptive RV remodeling in the setting of increased afterload (ie, pulmonary hypertension [PH]) will significantly affect TV function due to changes in the position of the papillary muscles (toward the apex), thus stretching of the tricuspid chordae leading to tenting or tethering of the leaflets, which results in leaflet malcoaptation.[17] More than mild TR is indeed predicted by end-systolic RV eccentricity index greater than 2.0 (area under the curve [AUC] 0.90), TV tethering area greater than 1.0 cm^2 (AUC 0.75), and end-diastolic TA diameter greater than 3.9 cm (AUC 0.65).[18] Recent studies however have shown that right atrial (RA) volume is a better predictor of TA area in secondary TR than RV end-diastolic volume, irrespective of cardiac rhythm and RV loading conditions.[19] This same study showed that the largest RA volume and smallest RV volumes were seen in patients with atrial fibrillation and secondary TR. Other studies confirm that atrial fibrillation is associated with larger RA volumes and TA areas in patients with TR[20] and is a predictor of TR progression along with an elevated pulmonary artery systolic pressure (PASP) of 36 mm Hg or greater.[21]

Given these clear morphologic differences, a more granular classification scheme has been developed, which not only includes differences in TV leaflet pathologic condition and mode of coaptation but also includes characteristic differences in TA, RV, and RA remodeling related to the distinct pathophysiology of secondary TR.[22,23]

CLASSIFICATION OF TRICUSPID REGURGITATION

The new classification scheme for TR challenges the simple classification of TR into primary disease defined as pathology of the leaflets, and secondary disease with intrinsically normal leaflets but abnormalities of the other TV apparatus. This classification scheme now recognizes the different morphologic entities of atrial and ventricular secondary TR, and a separate category of cardiac implantable electronic device (CIED)-related TR (**Table 1**).

Table 1
Classification of tricuspid regurgitation

Primary Tricuspid Regurgitation	Secondary Tricuspid Regurgitation	CIED-Related Tricuspid Regurgitation
Congenital 1. Ebstein anomaly 2. Atrioventricular canal defects 3. Tricuspid valve dysplasia	Atrial functional 1. Normal LV systolic function 2. Severe atrial dilatation 3. Absence of apical tethering of TV leaflets	CIED-induced leaflet impingement
Myxomatous degeneration	Ventricular functional due to left-sided disease 4. Left ventricular systolic dysfunction 5. Aortic valve disease 6. Mitral valve disease	
Systemic disease 1. Sarcoidosis 2. Lupus erythematosus 3. Rheumatic disease	Primary Right ventricular disease: 1) Right ventricular myopathy 2) RV ischemia 3)Arrhythmogenic right ventricular cardiomyopathy	
Malignancy 1. Carcinoid 2. Tumors involving right heart	Severe primary pulmonary hypertension	
Infective Endocarditis		
Iatrogenic causes 1. RV biopsy		
Chest wall trauma		
Drug induced		

Common causes of primary TR are shown in **Fig. 1**. Congenital causes of primary TR include: (1) Ebstein anomaly characterized by apical displacement of the TV leaflets, which originate from the RV with variable chordae resulting in atrialization of the RV; (2) atrioventricular canal resulting from failure of superior and inferior endocardium to fuse during embryologic development; and (3) TV dysplasia described as congenital malformation of the TV apparatus. In adults, the most common causes of primary TR include: (1) myxomatous degeneration of the TV; (2) systemic disease process including connective tissue disorders (sarcoidosis, lupus erythematosus, rheumatic disease); (3) infective endocarditis; (4) carcinogenic pathology (carcinoid, tumors involving right heart); (5) drug-induced inflammatory reaction (ergot derivatives, dopamine agonists, and anorectic medications); (6) chest wall trauma with injury to the RV and TV; and (7) trauma (biopsy or deceleration injury).

Although CIED leads have been classically categorized as a primary cause of TR, it is the device lead that has the direct effect on the leaflets or subvalvular apparatus and, thus, is considered a separate cause of TR.[24,25] CIED-induced TR may occur due to leaflet impingement by the lead without injury to the TV apparatus, or perforation of the leaflet, or adhesions/interference with the subvalvular apparatus (**Fig. 2**). CIED-induced is one of the most common causes of acquired TR with incidence of TR around 38% after lead placement.[26] CIED-induced TR is associated with a mortality of 10% to 20%.[27] The presence of a CIED is a strong predictor of progression of rapid progression og TR.[28] All-cause mortality (>1 year after pacemaker implantation) was higher in patients with TR deterioration (hazard ratio, 1.598; 95% CI, 1.275–2.002; $P < .01$).[25]

Ventricular secondary TR is characterized by dilatation, often in the midventricle resulting in a more spherical RV, RV dysfunction, and tethering of the TV leaflets. This cause is seen with pulmonary arterial hypertension, left-sided valvulopathy, and LV dysfunction.[29,30] Left-sided disease commonly results in pulmonary venous hypertension. Both pulmonary arterial, pulmonary venous, and mixed PH result in an increase in RV afterload and the cascade of adaptive and maladaptive changes resulting in TR (**Fig. 3**). Ventricular secondary TR in the presence of LV dysfunction (LVEF <50%), PH (PASP >50 mm Hg), and left-sided valvular disease carries a yearly mortality approaching 30%.[2]

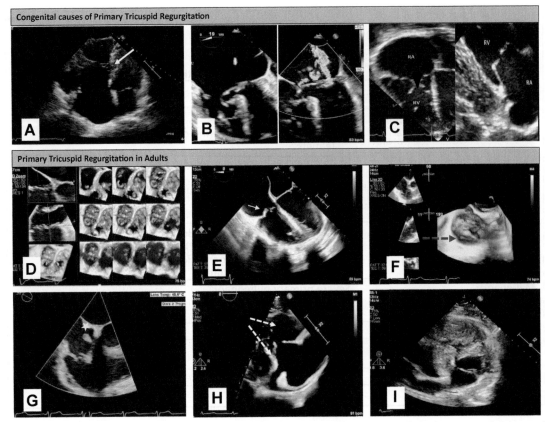

Fig. 1. Etiology of Primary TR. Congenital causes: (*A*) Ebstein anomaly with apical displacement of the septal leaflet (*white arrow*). (*B*) Atrio-ventricular canal defect. (*C*) Tricuspid atresia with abnormal development of the TV leaflets. Causes of Primary TR in adults (*D*) Prolapse: Multiplanar imaging showing short axis image of myxomatous TV with multileaflet thickening and prolapse. (*E*) Iatrogenic: Flail anterior leaflet (*yellow arrow*) following right heart biopsy. (*F*) Rheumatic disease of the TV with commissural fusion (*red dotted arrow*) (*G*) Endocarditis with vegetation on the atrial aspect of the anterior leaflet (*star*). (*H*) Carcinoid disease with thickened and fixed anterior and septal leaflets (*dotted white arrows*). (*I*) Angiosarcoma involving the RV.

Atrial secondary TR is characterized by less-prominent RV dilatation and therefore less TV leaflet tethering but marked dilatation of the TA and RA (**Fig. 3**).[31,32] Atrial functional TR is an increasingly recognized entity more so due to heightened awareness of atrial functional mitral regurgitation and its prognostic implications.[33,34] Recent studies have attempted to clearly define the clinical and morphologic characteristics of the disease. Based on a clustering approach, Schlotter and colleagues defined atrial secondary TR as TV tenting height of 10 mm or lesser, mid-ventricular RV diameter of 38 mm or lesser, and LV ejection fraction of 50% or greater.[35] Atrial secondary TR has a yearly mortality of only 10% to 15%.[2] In patients treated with transcatheter TV intervention (TTVI), atrial secondary TR was independently associated with a lower rate of the combined end point of mortality and heart failure hospitalization at 1-year follow-up (hazard ratio,

0.39; *P*<.05). Despite limited evidence to date, rhythm control may help to decrease atrial secondary TR in some patients through reverse remodeling of RA and TA.[36,37] Moreover, this form may be particularly amenable to treatment with annuloplasty devices because leaflet tethering is typically minimal.[19,38]

CLINICAL PRESENTATION

In the past, right-sided valvular disease and right heart failure have received less consideration from clinicians than left-sided disease. The heterogeneity of the disease process and its dependence with loading conditions, PH, hemodynamic alterations, rhythm abnormalities, comorbid conditions, and other contributing diseases have often confused care providers regarding the optimal timing of intervention. In the recent years, the focus has shifted to early identification and treatment

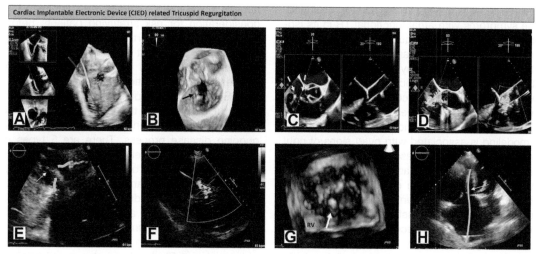

Fig. 2. CIED-related TR. (*A*) Septal-lateral and posterior trajectory of the pacemaker lead showing impingement of the posterior leaflet (*red arrow*). (*B*) Three-dimensional en face view showing pacemaker lead impingement at the level of the leaflet (*black arrow*). (*C*) Multiple pacemaker wires (*yellow dotted arrows*) noted crossing the TV annulus. (*D*) Regurgitant jets noted around both device wires. (*E*) Impingement of the subvalvular apparatus (*white arrow*). (*F*) regurgitant jet originating at the subvalvular level at the site of impingement. (*G*) Three-dimensional view from the RV showing subvalvular impingement (*white arrow*). (*H*) Septal trajectory taken by the distal end of the lead causing subvalvular impingement (*yellow arrow*).

because several studies have demonstrated the ominous impact of significant TR on mortality and morbidity with or without concomitant left-sided disease.[39,40]

Symptoms of TR are often nonspecific and covert. Due to the long latency period of severe TR, patients are referred for treatment during advanced stages. During the initial stages of the

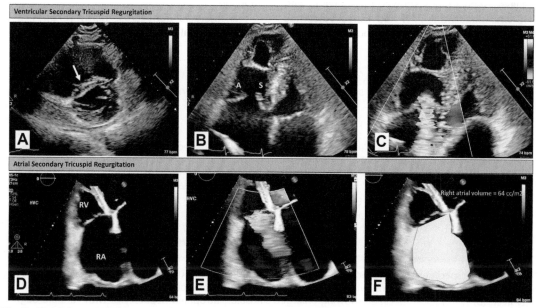

Fig. 3. Secondary TR (*A*) Severe right ventricular dilation with flattening of the interventricular septum (*white arrow*). (*B*) Apical tethering of the anterior and septal leaflet with large central coaptation gap. (*C*) Severe central TR. (*D*) Severe RA dilatation with RA larger than the RV. (*E*) Multiple regurgitant central jets. (*F*) RA volumetric assessment.

disease process, severe TR may be well tolerated. The symptoms with atrial functional TR in its isolated form are usually fatigue and exercise intolerance. This is due to poor cardiac output and loss of atrio-ventricular synchrony due to chronic atrial fibrillation. There is chronic elevation of RA pressure, which may result in congestive hepatopathy and signs of venous congestion.

Conversely, a long-standing TR or TR with RV remodeling is associated with overt signs of right heart failure resulting in ascites, loss of appetite, hepatic dysfunction, and anasarca. Cardiohepatic syndrome (CHS) is often noted in patients with chronic TR with persistently elevated RA pressures. CHS is mainly classified into 2 types. Type I CHS is seen in acute decompensated heart failure resulting in hypoxic or ischemic hepatitis and shock liver. This results in hepatocellular death either due to hypoperfusion and necrosis (elevated transaminases) or cholestasis due to systemic congestion (elevated bilirubin, alkaline phosphatase, and gamma glutamyl transferase). Type 2 CHS is associated with chronic heart failure and is often referred to as congestive hepatopathy. This results in sinusoidal dilatation commonly referred to as nut meg liver on histological examination (**Fig. 4**). Transaminases in this population are usually within the reference range with elevated levels of bilirubin, alkaline phosphatase, and gamma glutamyl transferase.[41] Biventricular failure may lead to microcirculatory dysfunction and cellular cytolysis and elevated level of transaminase. Recent study showed that patients with CHS who underwent TTVI had worse outcomes when compared with those without.[42] Degree of

hepatic impairment should be an important consideration for risk stratifying patients before intervention and all efforts must be made to recognize hepatic decline at an early stage when TV intervention may lead to hepatic regeneration and restoration of function.

CHS is often accompanied by cardiorenal syndrome (CRS). CRS is the interaction of cardiac and renal function and vice-versa during an ongoing disease process. There are 5 types of CRS: types 1 and 2 reflect the impact of acute and chronic diseases of the heart, respectively, on the renal function and vice versa, the effects of acute and chronic diseases of the kidney on the heart are classified as types 3 and 4, respectively. Type 5 is concomitant impact on both organs due to a common systemic illness effecting both organs.[43] Studies have shown reduction in abdominal congestion and stable or reduction in diuretic doses after TTVI; however, improvement in renal function after intervention was not demonstrated.[44–46]

ROLE OF IMAGING IN TRICUSPID REGURGITATION

In the era of emerging new therapies for management of TV disease, multimodality imaging plays a crucial role in preprocedural, intraprocedural, and postprocedural assessments. Imaging plays a vital role in identifying and differentiating the mechanism of TR as well as the assessment of right heart function.

Transthoracic Echocardiography (TTE): TTE is the ideal initial imaging modality and serves to

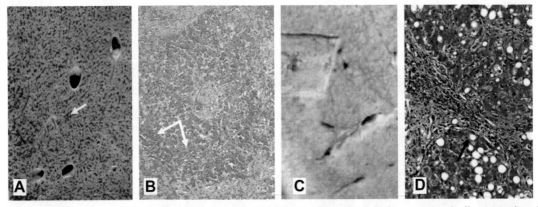

Fig. 4. (*A*) Gross specimen showing reddish central areas that represent sinusoidal congestion (*yellow arrow*) and bleeding in the atrophied regions, with contrasting yellowish discoloration representing either normal liver or fatty liver. (*B*) Histological specimen showing enlarged sinusoids, atrophied hepatocytes with variable degrees of hemorrhage (*white arrows*). (*C*) Gross specimen from alcoholic cirrhosis showing nodularity. Cirrhosis due to other causes often results in the loss of normal lobular architecture of hepatic parenchyma and replacement with regenerative nodules and fibrous tissue. (*D*) Histological specimen showing fibrous septa that divide the hepatic parenchyma into nodules (*black arrow*).

establish the diagnosis. TTE besides being an easily accessible, noninvasive modality with high temporal resolution is unique in its ability to image the TV and the right heart. Due to the proximity of the right heart to chest wall owing to the anterior position, TV is a near field structure and imaging from parasternal views provides excellent anatomical and functional evaluation.[47] The primary objectives of the echocardiogram are as follows:

1. Define TV anatomy
2. Determine the cause of TR
3. Assess the severity of TR by both qualitative and quantitative methods
4. Characterize right ventricular and RA anatomy and function
5. Assess for other associated valvular pathologic condition and left-sided function
6. Image extracardiac structures—inferior vena cava (IVC) and superior vena cava (SVC)
7. Assess flow pattern of the hepatic vein
8. Evaluate feasibility of TV intervention

Tricuspid Valve Assessment: Due to the complexity of TV apparatus, multiple views should be used for imaging the TV leaflets, annulus and subvalvular apparatus. Ideally, both two-dimensional (2D) and three-dimensional (3D) imaging should be performed from multiple imaging windows to assess the anatomy. Off-axis imaging may be needed in patients where there is a massive RV or RA dilation. Recent studies have shed light on the variability in the number of TV leaflets, and efforts are underway to standardize the nomenclature of TV.[10] Evaluation of leaflet integrity and structure is critical while considering patients for TTVI. Three-dimensional imaging from transthoracic windows is often equivalent or better than TEE images due to the proximity of the probe to the valve. Narrow sector volumes focused on the valve from multiple views should be acquired.[48] Multibeat acquisition improves the frame rate and allows for direct planimetry of the regurgitant orifice area also known as vena contracta area. The approach to comprehensive assessment of the TV is addressed in the American Society of Echocardiography guidelines.[49,50]

Right Ventricular Assessment: Presence of concomitant right ventricular dysfunction with TR is considered high risk for any kind of TV intervention.[51,52] The vicious cycle of TR and right heart dysfunction is driven by the valvular pathologic condition. Progressive right heart failure often manifests as systemic venous congestion (edema, ascites), organ dysfunction (liver, kidney, bowel), and coagulopathy (hepatic and splenic dysfunction). Thorough assessment of RV function is critical at the time of TR assessment to help

improve patient selection and determine optimal timing of intervention.

The conventional independent echocardiographic parameters used for the assessment of RV are tricuspid annular plane systolic excursion (TAPSE), fractional area change (FAC), RV myocardial performance index, lateral annulus peak systolic velocity (RV S′), and RV dP/dt. The comprehensive assessment of RV using these parameters is described in the ASE guidelines.[49] Newer echocardiographic methods of assessing RV function include RV strain, either free wall or global (including the septum)[53,54] and 3D RV ejection fraction[55,56] have been increasingly used clinically and have been associated with outcomes in patients with severe TR.[57–59]

In a compensated state, the RV adapts by increase in contractility with increasing afterload, whereas in decompensated state, RV function fails to increase. The assessment of RV contractile performance against the afterload by determining RV–PA coupling ratios provides important information regarding compensatory state of the RV and is a valuable prognostic marker in patients with HF with reduced ore preserved ejection fraction, PH as well as any valvular dysfunction.[60–64] The RV–PA coupling ratio is determined noninvasively by the ratio of TAPSE and echocardiographically derived PASP. TAPSE/PASP is associated with outcomes in patients with untreated secondary TR[65] as well as patients undergoing TTVI.[66] Recent analysis of the data from the TriValve registry also showed that patients whose RV–PA coupling ratio declined following TTVI had a better outcome compared with patients whose ratio did not change, suggesting that RV reserve may also be an important prognostic marker when considering TV intervention.[66]

Pulmonary Vascular Assessment: PH often co-exists with significant TR and is associated with adverse outcomes following TV intervention.[18] Evaluation of baseline PASP is used to determine the preoperative risk. Echocardiographically determined PASP does not always correlate with invasive measurement, and therefore, combining invasive and echocardiographic PH assessment is necessary for preprocedural risk stratification. Recent study has shown that subjects with discordant invasive and echocardiographic PH have worst outcomes following TTVI.[67,68] Echocardiographic parameters for RV assessment are summarized in **Fig. 5**.

Transesophageal echocardiogram (TEE): TEE examination done at various levels and multiplane angles allows for complete visualization and assessment of the TV apparatus and the RV. Additionally, careful assessment and quantification of

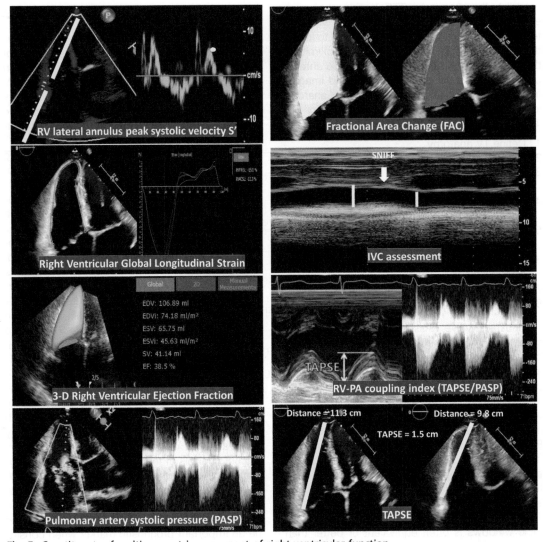

Fig. 5. Constituents of multiparametric assessment of right ventricular function.

left-sided pathologic condition, which may be contributing to this disease process, is also feasible. Visualization of the TV can be sometimes challenging by TEE in patients with horizontal heart, left-sided prosthesis, lipomatous interatrial septum, or atrial septal devices due to acoustic shadowing of the TV leaflets because the ultrasound beam crosses these structures. Although imaging from the midesophageal level, the esophagus is further away from the TV. Imaging from the distal esophagus and the stomach allows for cleaner views of the TV because it is closer to the esophagus and hence the imaging probe. The guidelines for performing TEE by American Society of Echocardiography outline the key views for imaging the TV.[69,70] Ability to visualize the TV leaflets, subvalvular apparatus, and surrounding landmarks is crucial for TTVI. Three-dimensional

imaging allows for careful delineation of the TV leaflets, aides in understanding the pathologic condition and allows for planning the interventional procedures.

The key views for TV and right heart evaluation by TTE and TEE are summarized in **Figs. 6** and **7** respectively.

Intracardiac Imaging (ICE): ICE catheter is a narrow 3.0-mm tip (9 French) catheter that is introduced via the femoral vein and navigated to the heart for acquisition of high-quality 2D and 3D images in real-time. ICE during intraprocedural imaging is often used to supplement TEE imaging during transcatheter procedures. Acoustic shadowing from the delivery system or the prosthesis itself may lead to drop out with TEE imaging. ICE provides incremental value in such circumstances. The currently available 4D ICE catheters can

Key Transthoracic Views	Pictorial Depiction	Structures Imaged
Parasternal RV inflow	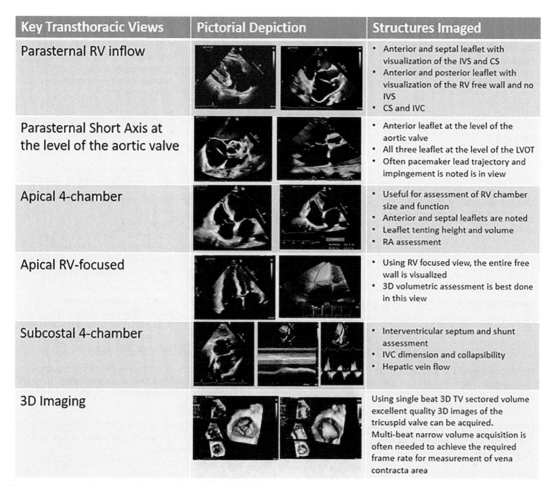	• Anterior and septal leaflet with visualization of the IVS and CS • Anterior and posterior leaflet with visualization of the RV free wall and no IVS • CS and IVC
Parasternal Short Axis at the level of the aortic valve		• Anterior leaflet at the level of the aortic valve • All three leaflet at the level of the LVOT • Often pacemaker lead trajectory and impingement is noted is in view
Apical 4-chamber		• Useful for assessment of RV chamber size and function • Anterior and septal leaflets are noted • Leaflet tenting height and volume • RA assessment
Apical RV-focused		• Using RV focused view, the entire free wall is visualized • 3D volumetric assessment is best done in this view
Subcostal 4-chamber		• Interventricular septum and shunt assessment • IVC dimension and collapsibility • Hepatic vein flow
3D Imaging		Using single beat 3D TV sectored volume excellent quality 3D images of the tricuspid valve can be acquired. Multi-beat narrow volume acquisition is often needed to achieve the required frame rate for measurement of vena contracta area

Fig. 6. Key views for transthoracic imaging of the TV.

obtain 2D and 3D volumetric images and cine-videos in real-time (4D) (**Fig. 8**). ICE has been proven to be a safe and efficacious modality for transcatheter electrophysiological as well as structural heart interventions.[71] Although currently used to complement the TEE imaging, in the future ICE may be used as a standalone device for imaging during TTVI.[72–75]

Multidetector Computed Tomography (MDCT): Specific acquisition protocols are needed for optimized imaging of the right heart and TV by MDCT. Type of scanner, left ventricular function, heart rate, presence of arrhythmia, renal function, and body habitus are key elements that should be accounted for while designing patient-specific protocol for the assessment of TR. Triphasic contrast bolus with contrast, mixture of saline/contrast and saline should be used.[76] Multiphasic cardiac-gated acquisition with imaging throughout the cardiac cycle must be attained to allow for postacquisition reconstruction from different phases. Cine imaging allows for the dynamic

assessment of RV. Higher temporal resolution is achieved with dual source scanners or using multi-beat acquisition with a single source scanner. RV volumes and function can be analyzed by semiautomated segmentation of the RV throughout the cardiac cycle. All 3 modalities have been shown to have excellent correlation in the assessment of RV function and volume.[77,78]

MDCT can provide characterization and precise measurements of the TA that help in sizing for TTVR. High temporal and spatial resolution also allow for the assessment of number of leaflets, delineation of TR cause (primary vs secondary), degree of prolapse/flail, extent of leaflet tenting, coaptation gap, as well as assessment of RA and RV chamber size (**Fig. 9**). Characterization of sub-valvular apparatus and RV length and trabeculations are crucial to planning valvular intervention because certain devices need anchoring or clearance in the RV before deployment of the prosthesis. Retrograde opacification of IVC and hepatic veins with iodinated contrast is a specific

Key Transesophageal Views	Pictorial Depiction	Structures Imaged
Mid-esophageal 4-chamber at 0° rotation		• Anterior and septal leaflet morphology and length • Coaptation gap • Measurement of vena contracta • Measurement of TA
Mid-esophageal TV commissural view at 60°– 90°		• Anterior leaflet and posterior leaflet at the level of the aortic valve • Pacemaker lead trajectory and its position • Alignment to jet for doppler assessment (CW and PW at annulus)
Mid-esophageal TV commissural view at 60°– 90° with orthogonal biplane imaging		• Useful for assessment of leaflet integrity • Biplane sweep view allows for assessment of leaflet morphology sweeping from A-S to P-S leaflets • Assessment of jet width and extent • Key view for procedural guidance for TTVI
Deep esophageal 0°		• Here TV is in close proximity to the probe and in cases of left sided prosthesis deep esophageal views may be used for complete assessment including 3D images
Deep esophageal RV inflow outflow view at 60° — 90°		• Like ME views this helps in assessment of number of jets and leaflet morphology
Trans gastric short axis view of the TV at 30°–60°		Important view for assessing number of leaflets Presence of cleft and assessment of commissures Measurement of coaptation gaps Procedural guidance for TTVI
3D Imaging		Leaflet characterization 3D annular measurement for device sizing 3D Vena contracta measurement 3D planimetry of valve area at leaflet tips

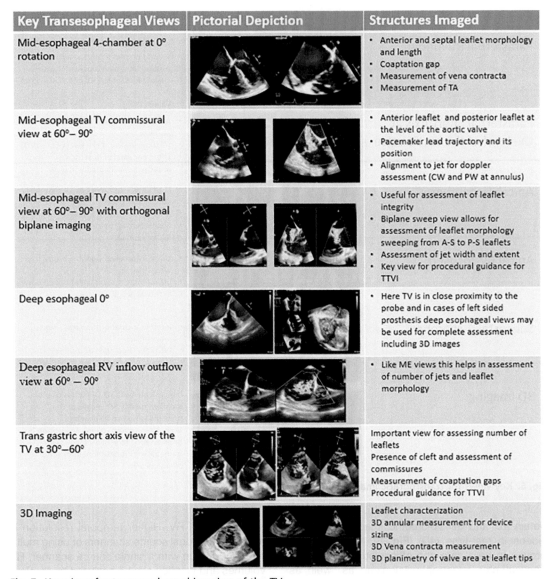

Fig. 7. Key views for transesophageal imaging of the TV.

marker of right heart disease and is often noted in patients with severe TR.[79] Unique to this modality is the benefit of planning of procedure by visualization of abdominal vasculature and access; accurate location and course of the right coronary artery in relation to the TA and assessment of the angulation between the IVC and TV.[80] Motion and misintegration artifact are often seen in patients with atrial fibrillation. Newer generation multidetector scanners allow for shorter scan times and are less prone to artifact. Patient-specific protocol planning is key for acquiring the best possible dataset for comprehensive assessment of right heart pathologic condition.

Cardiac Magnetic Resonance (CMR): Accurate and reproducible assessment of RV function,

wall motion abnormality, RV volume, and chamber quantification can be accomplished by CMR.[81,82] CMR plays a unique role in identifying right ventricular remodeling and fibrosis without the use of ionizing radiation. This imaging modality is the gold standard for tissue characterization. RV tissue characterization is possible using native T1 imaging and delayed gadolinium enhancement. Myocarditis, myocardial infarction, infiltrative disease, trauma, as well as PH can be differentiated using this modality. Regurgitant volume and regurgitant fraction for quantitative assessment of TR can be done using right-sided chamber volume along with phase contrast pulmonic flow. Short-axis cine images are typically used for volumetric measurements by tracing endocardial borders

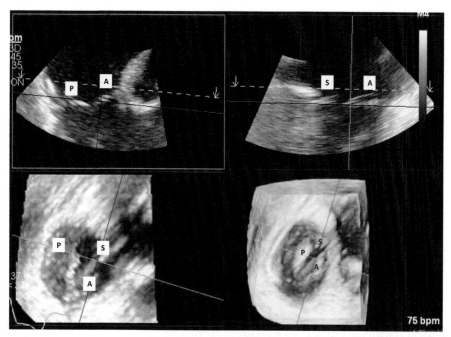

Fig. 8. Three-dimensional volumetric image of TV in real time using ICE catheter for procedural guidance.

using semiautomated tracing techniques (see **Fig. 9**). Similar to MDCT, imaging protocols should account for the dilation of the RV and right atrium and include 4-chamber, RV inflow–outflow, and RV short axis images in its entirety. Leaflet length,

tenting, prolapse, and thickening can all be assessed using sequential thin slice imaging.

CMR may be limited by arrhythmias, which often lead to motion artifact. Real-time cine imaging without breath-hold instructions are used in the

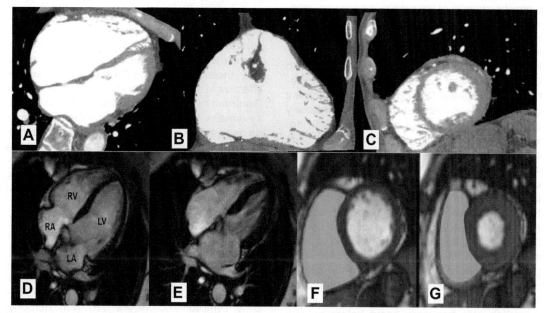

Fig. 9. Assessment of the RV using CT and MRI. (*A–C*) Anatomical assessment of the RV in multiple planes. (*D, E*) RV FAC assessment with MRI. (*F, G*) Endocardial tracing of short-axis cine images for the volumetric assessment of RV function.

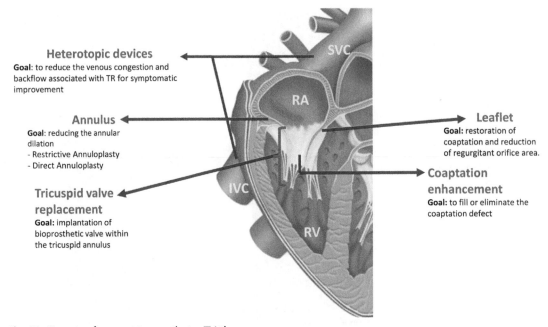

Heterotopic devices
Goal: to reduce the venous congestion and
backflow associated with TR for symptomatic
improvement

SVC

RA

Leaflet
Goal: restoration of
coaptation and reduction
of regurgitant orifice area.

Annulus
Goal: reducing the annular
dilation
- Restrictive Annuloplasty
- Direct Annuloplasty

IVC

**Coaptation
enhancement**
Goal: to fill or eliminate the
coaptation defect

**Tricuspid valve
replacement**
Goal: implantation of
bioprosthetic valve within
the tricuspid annulus

RV

Fig. 10. Targets of current transcatheter TV therapy.

patients with arrhythmia; however, the image resolution in such cases is suboptimal. Shortened
free breathing real-time acquisition may be used
to offset this problem. Presence of prosthetic devices and pacemaker leads may induce artifacts
due to local magnetic field inhomogeneities. The
interference of the magnetic field with the ferromagnetic material of the cardiac device may inad-
vertently lead to dislocation or loss of function.
Historically, the presence of intracardiac device
was considered as a contraindication to CMR.
However, efforts are underway to transition to
CMR-safe devices that have less interaction between the magnetic field due to reduced amount
of ferromagnetic material from the previously
available CMR-conditional and CMR-unsafe devices. CMR conditional pacemakers have been
commercially available since 2011 and majority
of the patient population we deal with have these
devices. The devices should be reprogrammed
to prevent inappropriate activation or shock, and
typically, CMR sequences with a specific absorption rate of 2.0 W/kg or lesser should be used.[83]
Several techniques have been developed to avoid
image artifacts, these include the use of imaging
planes perpendicular to the plane of the cardiac
device, inversion and excitation pulses bandwidth
widening, echo time shortening, and the imple-
mentation of a frequency scout before steady-
state free precession sequences or the use of
spoiled gradient echo cine imaging.[84–86]

NOVEL TREATMENT STRATEGIES

Current guideline-directed medical treatment includes a IIa recommendation for diuretics, aimed
at reducing the preload; however, the level of evidence (Category C) remains limited.[3] Guidelines
also give a IIa recommendation for the treatment
of left heart disease and PH, which is aimed at
reducing the afterload. Although the evidence is
also limited for this recommendation, recent
studies suggest that the reduction of mitral regurgitation with TEER[87] and cardiac resynchronization therapy for left heart failure[88] may be
effective in reducing TR and improving outcomes.
Recurrent heart failure hospitalizations and mortality remains high despite medical therapy. Based
on degree of regurgitation and presence of symptoms various stages of TR have been defined by
the recent The American College of Cardiology
and American Heart Association (ACC/AHA)
guidelines for the management of valvular heart
disease.

Stage B represents progressive TR, quantified as nonsevere without any hemodynamic
consequences. Stage C is asymptomatic severe TR with hemodynamic consequences like
dilated RA/RV with elevated right sided pressures, but no patient reported symptoms. Stage
D is symptomatic severe TR, with hemodynamic consequences and patient reported
symptoms.

Table 2
Current devices under investigation for transcatheter tricuspid valve intervention

Device Target	Current Devices	Useful Imaging Modalities	Advantages	Limitations
Annulus Goal: reducing the annular dilation	Restrictive Annuloplasty • TRIAPTA (transatrial intrapericardial tricuspid annuloplasty) Direct Annuloplasty • Cardioband (Edwards Lifesciences) • MIA-T (Micro Interventional Devices, Inc) • DaVingi (Cardiac Implants LLC)	Baseline: CT • Annular sizing - location of RCA TEE for baseline annular sizing and quantification of regurgitation and chamber dimensions Intraprocedural: TEE and ICE for intraprocedural guidance Postprocedure: TTE and CT for postprocedural follow-up	Useful for regurgitation due to annular dilation Useful in atrial functional TR	• In investigational stages • Challenges with anchor deployment along the ill-defined tricuspid annulus • Proximity of the RCA to the annulus may prove to be a limitation
Leaflet Goal: restoration of coaptation and reduction of regurgitant orifice area	• TriClip (Abbott Vascular, Santa Clara, Ca) • PASCAL (Edwards Lifesciences)	Baseline: TTE and TEE: For quantification of regurgitation and assessment of leaflet morphology and coaptation gaps. CT may also be helpful in measurement of coaptation gap Intraprocedural: TEE and ICE for intraprocedural guidance Postprocedure: TTE with 3D assessment of prosthesis	• Most experience among tricuspid devices • No need for full anticoagulation postimplantation unlike valve replacement	• Procedural learning curve • Incomplete reduction of TR • Not ideal for regurgitation with large central coaptation gaps • Not ideal for multiple regurgitant jets
Coaptation enhancement Goal: to fill or eliminate the coaptation defect	• DUO • TriFlo	TEE/CT or MRI	• Ideal for patients with large central coaptation defects	

(continued on next page)

Table 2
(continued)

Device Target	Current Devices	Useful Imaging Modalities	Advantages	Limitations
TV replacement Goal: implantation of bioprosthetic valve within the tricuspid annulus	• EVOQUE system (Edwards Lifesciences) • LuX-Valve (Ningbo Jenscare Biotechnology, China) • Intrepid (Medtronic) • Tricares • Trisol • V-Dyne • Cardiovalve	Baseline: TEE/TTE: For quantification of regurgitation and assessment of leaflet morphology and annular measurement. RV assessment CT is mainstay for annular measurement and sizing Intraprocedural: TEE and ICE for intraprocedural guidance Postprocedure: TTE with 3D assessment of prosthesis. CT for prosthetic valve dysfunction and RV assessment	• Complete elimination of TR • Ideal for patients with large coaptation gaps	• Limited data on long-term durability • Management of RV dysfunction postprocedure may be challenging • It is unclear who the ideal candidates for this therapy would be
Heterotopic devices Goal: to reduce the venous congestion and backflow associated with TR for symptomatic improvement	• TricValve (P&F products Features Vertriebs, Vienna, Austria) • Tricento (NVT GmBH Hechingen, Germany) • Caval SAPIEN 3 (Edwards Lifesciences)	Baseline: CT: Measurement of the IVC and SVC dimensions Intraprocedural: TEE and TTE: To assess landing zones of the valves Fluoroscopy is used as adjunctive imaging Postprocedure: TTE	• May be the only option currently available for patients with severe annular dilatation who do not make the inclusion criteria for TTVR and have large coaptation gaps, which make them poor candidate for TEER therapy	• Little or no effect on immediate right heart hemodynamics • Cannot be used for patients with severe caval enlargement

TR Patient's Journey

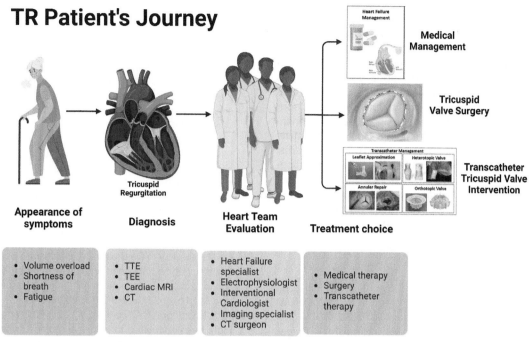

Fig. 11. Clinical journey of patient presenting with TR. (*Created with* BioRender.com.)

Both ACC/AHA guidelines and ESC/EACTS guidelines[89] recommend surgical intervention for severe primary or secondary TR at the time of left-sided intervention for patients with Stage C or D (Class I) and to prevent the progression of secondary disease in Stage B patients who exhibit TA dilatation of more than 4 cm and/or RV dysfunction (Class IIa). TV surgery for isolated primary TR received a IIa indication for Stage D and IIb for Stage C. Patients with secondary TR attributable to annular dilatation (without PH or left-sided disease) who are poorly responsive to medical therapy, TV surgery is a Class IIa indication. Surgery however was favored in the ESC and EACTS recommendations that gave it a Class 1 for isolated severe primary TR without severe RV dysfunction.[89]

The key to ensure positive outcomes is patient selection. Severely reduced RV function, congestive hepatopathy, and multiorgan dysfunction often are markers for poor outcomes. The advent of transcatheter therapy is a promising new approach to manage this challenging patient population. The targets of current TV therapy are demonstrated in **Fig. 10**. The treatment of severe TR with transcatheter edge-to-edge repair (TEER) therapy is recognized as 2b recommendation by 2021 ESC/ECATS due to Conformité Européene approved tricuspid TEER device in inoperable patients at a comprehensive heart center with expertise. The current devices under investigation are listed in **Table 2**.

There are several challenges with designing trials for the treatment of TV disease using minimally invasive transcatheter approach. Standardization of patient selection criteria based on preprocedural imaging and clinical assessment is needed to warrant positive outcomes. Identifying goals of therapy upfront is critical and would play a crucial role in device selection. Ideal timing of intervention to ensure best possible outcomes is yet to be defined. Early recognition, referral, and timely intervention may prevent the progression to refractory right heart failure, RV chamber dilation, and end-organ dysfunction (**Fig. 11**).

CLINICS CARE POINTS

- Before consideration of invasive intervention, optimization of hemodynamic state has shown to improve outcomes.

- In the presence of CIED, look for device impingement on the TV apparatus.

- Involve heart failure team right from the time of initial assessment and diagnosis.

DISCLOSURE

Dr V Agarwal reports speaker fees from Abbott Structural; she has a consulting agreement with ReNiva Inc. and Moray medical. Dr R. Hahn reports speaker fees from Abbott Structural, Baylis Medical, Edwards Lifesciences, and Philips Healthcare; she has institutional consulting contracts for which she receives no direct compensation with Abbott Structural, Boston Scientific, Edwards Lifesciences, Medtronic and Novartis; she is Chief Scientific Officer for the Echocardiography Core Laboratory at the Cardiovascular Research Foundation for multiple industry-sponsored TV trials, for which she receives no direct industry compensation.

REFERENCES

1. Dreyfus GD, Martin RP, Chan KM, et al. Functional tricuspid regurgitation: a need to revise our understanding. J Am Coll Cardiol 2015;65:2331–6.

2. Topilsky Y, Maltais S, Medina Inojosa J, et al. Burden of Tricuspid Regurgitation in Patients Diagnosed in the Community Setting. JACC Cardiovasc Imaging 2019;12:433–42.

3. Otto CM, Nishimura RA, Bonow RO, et al. 2020 ACC/AHA Guideline for the Management of Patients With Valvular Heart Disease: A Report of the American College of Cardiology/American Heart Association Joint, Committee on Clinical Practice Guidelines. J Am Coll Cardiol 2021;77:e25–197.

4. Dahou A, Levin D, Reisman M, et al. Anatomy and Physiology of the Tricuspid Valve. JACC Cardiovasc Imaging 2019;12:458–68.

5. Addetia K, Muraru D, Veronesi F, et al. 3-Dimensional Echocardiographic Analysis of the Tricuspid Annulus Provides New Insights Into Tricuspid Valve Geometry and Dynamics. J Am Coll Cardiol 2017; 12(3):401–12.

6. Messer S, Moseley E, Marinescu M, et al. Histologic analysis of the right atrioventricular junction in the adult human heart. J Heart Valve Dis 2012;21:368–73.

7. El-Busaid H, Hassan S, Odula P, et al. Sex variations in the structure of human atrioventricular annuli. Folia Morphol (Warsz) 2012;71:23–7.

8. Singh JP, Evans JC, Levy D, et al. Prevalence and clinical determinants of mitral, tricuspid, and aortic regurgitation (the Framingham Heart Study). Am J Cardiol 1999;83:897–902.

9. Naser JA, Pislaru C, Roslan A, et al. Unfavorable Tricuspid Annulus Dynamics: A Novel Concept to Explain Development of Tricuspid Regurgitation in Atrial Fibrillation. J Am Soc Echocardiogr 2022;35: 664–6.

10. Hahn RT, Weckbach LT, Noack T, et al. Proposal for a Standard Echocardiographic Tricuspid Valve Nomenclature. JACC Cardiovasc Imaging 2021; 14(7):1299–305.

11. Haddad F, Hunt SA, Rosenthal DN, et al. Right ventricular function in cardiovascular disease, part I: Anatomy, physiology, aging, and functional assessment of the right ventricle. Circulation 2008;117:1436–48.

12. Sanz J, Sánchez-Quintana D, Bossone E, et al. Anatomy, Function, and Dysfunction of the Right Ventricle: JACC State-of-the-Art Review. J Am Coll Cardiol 2019;73:1463–82.

13. MacNee W. Pathophysiology of cor pulmonale in chronic obstructive pulmonary disease. Part One. Am J Respir Crit Care Med 1994;150:833–52.

14. Bartelds B, Borgdorff MA, Smit-van Oosten A, et al. Differential responses of the right ventricle to abnormal loading conditions in mice: pressure vs. volume load. Eur J Heart Fail 2011;13:1275–82.

15. De Meester P, Van De Bruaene A, Herijgers P, et al. Geometry of the right heart and tricuspid regurgitation to exclude elevated pulmonary artery pressure: new insights. Int J Cardiol 2013;168:3866–71.

16. Vonk-Noordegraaf A, Haddad F, Chin KM, et al. Right heart adaptation to pulmonary arterial hypertension: physiology and pathobiology. J Am Coll Cardiol 2013;62:D22–33.

17. Spinner EM, Lerakis S, Higginson J, et al. Correlates of tricuspid regurgitation as determined by 3D echocardiography: pulmonary arterial pressure, ventricle geometry, annular dilatation, and papillary muscle displacement. Circ Cardiovasc Imaging 2012;5:43–50.

18. Kim YJ, Kwon DA, Kim HK, et al. Determinants of surgical outcome in patients with isolated tricuspid regurgitation. Circulation 2009;120:1672–8.

19. Muraru D, Addetia K, Guta AC, et al. Right atrial volume is a major determinant of tricuspid annulus area in functional tricuspid regurgitation: a three-dimensional echocardiographic study. Eur Heart J Cardiovasc Imaging 2021;22:660–9.

20. Utsunomiya H, Itabashi Y, Mihara H, et al. Functional Tricuspid Regurgitation Caused by Chronic Atrial Fibrillation: A Real-Time 3-Dimensional Transesophageal Echocardiography Study. Circ Cardiovasc Imaging 2017;10.

21. Mutlak D, Khalil J, Lessick J, et al. Risk Factors for the Development of Functional Tricuspid Regurgitation and Their Population-Attributable Fractions. JACC Cardiovasc Imaging 2020;13:1643–51.

22. Praz F, Muraru D, Kreidel F, et al. Transcatheter treatment for tricuspid valve disease. EuroIntervention 2021;17:791–808.

23. Lancellotti P, Pibarot P, Chambers J, et al. Multi-modality imaging assessment of native valvular regurgitation: an EACVI and ESC council of valvular heart disease position paper. Eur Heart J Cardiovasc Imaging 2022;23(5):e171–232.

24. Addetia K, Harb SC, Hahn RT, et al. Cardiac Implantable Electronic Device Lead-Induced

Tricuspid Regurgitation. JACC Cardiovasc Imaging 2019;12:622–36.

25. Zhang XX, Wei M, Xiang R, et al. Incidence, Risk Factors, and Prognosis of Tricuspid Regurgitation After Cardiac Implantable Electronic Device Implantation: A Systematic Review and Meta-analysis. J Cardiothorac Vasc Anesth 2022;36:1741–55.

26. Hoke U, Auger D, Thijssen J, et al. Significant lead-induced tricuspid regurgitation is associated with poor prognosis at long-term follow-up. Heart 2014; 100:960–8.

27. Delling FN, Hassan ZK, Piatkowski G, et al. Tricuspid Regurgitation and Mortality in Patients With Transvenous Permanent Pacemaker Leads. Am J Cardiol 2016;117:988–92.

28. Prihadi EA, van der Bijl P, Gursoy E, et al. Development of significant tricuspid regurgitation over time and prognostic implications: new insights into natural history. Eur Heart J 2018;39:3574–81.

29. Arsalan M, Walther T, Smith RL 2nd, et al. Tricuspid regurgitation diagnosis and treatment. Eur Heart J 2017;38:634–8.

30. Badano LP, Muraru D, Enriquez-Sarano M. Assessment of functional tricuspid regurgitation. Eur Heart J 2013;34:1875–85.

31. Muraru D, Guta AC, Ochoa-Jimenez RC, et al. Functional Regurgitation of Atrioventricular Valves and Atrial Fibrillation: An Elusive Pathophysiological Link Deserving Further Attention. J Am Soc Echocardiogr 2020;33:42–53.

32. Florescu DR, Muraru D, Volpato V, et al. Atrial Functional Tricuspid Regurgitation as a Distinct Pathophysiological and Clinical Entity: No Idiopathic Tricuspid Regurgitation Anymore. J Clin Med 2022; 11:382.

33. Delgado V, Bax JJ. Atrial Functional Mitral Regurgitation: From Mitral Annulus Dilatation to Insufficient Leaflet Remodeling. Circ Cardiovasc Imaging 2017;10:e006239.

34. Zoghbi WA, Levine RA, Flachskampf F, et al. Atrial Functional Mitral Regurgitation: A JACC: Cardiovascular Imaging Expert Panel Viewpoint. JACC Cardiovasc Imaging 2022;15:1870–82.

35. Schlotter F, Dietz MF, Stolz L, et al. Atrial Functional Tricuspid Regurgitation: Novel Definition and Impact on Prognosis. Circ Cardiovasc Interv 2022;15: e011958.

36. Vahanian A, Beyersdorf F, Praz F, et al. 2021 ESC/EACTS Guidelines for the management of valvular heart disease: Developed by the Task Force for the management of valvular heart disease of the European Society of Cardiology (ESC) and the European Association for Cardio-Thoracic Surgery (EACTS). Eur Heart J 2021;75(6):524.

37. Muraru D, Caravita S, Guta AC, et al. Functional Tricuspid Regurgitation and Atrial Fibrillation: Which

Comes First, the Chicken or the Egg? CASE (Philadelphia, Pa) 2020;4:458–63.

38. Badano LP, Caravita S, Rella V, et al. The Added Value of 3-Dimensional Echocardiography to Understand the Pathophysiology of Functional Tricuspid Regurgitation. JACC Cardiovasc Imaging 2021;14: 683–9.

39. Topilsky Y, Inojosa JM, Benfari G, et al. Clinical presentation and outcome of tricuspid regurgitation in patients with systolic dysfunction. Eur Heart J 2018;39:3584–92.

40. Topilsky Y, Nkomo VT, Vatury O, et al. Clinical outcome of isolated tricuspid regurgitation. JACC Cardiovasc Imaging 2014;7:1185–94.

41. Poelzl G, Auer J. Cardiohepatic syndrome. Curr Heart Fail Rep 2015;12:68–78.

42. Stolz L, Orban M, Besler C, et al. Cardiohepatic Syndrome Is Associated With Poor Prognosis in Patients Undergoing Tricuspid Transcatheter Edge-to-Edge Valve Repair. JACC Cardiovasc Interv 2022;15: 179–89.

43. House AA, Anand I, Bellomo R, et al. Definition and classification of Cardio-Renal Syndromes: workgroup statements from the 7th ADQI Consensus Conference. Nephrol Dial Transplant 2010;25: 1416–20.

44. Hewing B, Mattig I, Knebel F, et al. Renal and hepatic function of patients with severe tricuspid regurgitation undergoing inferior caval valve implantation. Sci Rep 2021;11:21800.

45. Lauten A, Figulla HR, Unbehaun A, et al. Interventional Treatment of Severe Tricuspid Regurgitation: Early Clinical Experience in a Multicenter, Observational, First-in-Man Study. Circ Cardiovasc Interv 2018;11:e006061.

46. Karam N, Braun D, Mehr M, et al. Impact of Transcatheter Tricuspid Valve Repair for Severe Tricuspid Regurgitation on Kidney and Liver Function. JACC Cardiovasc Interv 2019;12:1413–20.

47. Lancellotti P, Tribouilloy C, Hagendorff A, et al. Recommendations for the echocardiographic assessment of native valvular regurgitation: an executive summary from the European Association of Cardiovascular Imaging. Eur Heart J Cardiovasc Imaging 2013;14:611–44.

48. Muraru D, Hahn RT, Soliman OI, et al. 3-Dimensional Echocardiography in Imaging the Tricuspid Valve. JACC Cardiovasc Imaging 2019;12:500–15.

49. Rudski LG, Lai WW, Afilalo J, et al. Guidelines for the echocardiographic assessment of the right heart in adults: a report from the American Society of Echocardiography endorsed by the European Association of Echocardiography, a registered branch of the European Society of Cardiology, and the Canadian Society of Echocardiography. J Am Soc Echocardiogr 2010;23:685–713 [quiz: 786–8].

50. Lang RM, Badano LP, Tsang W, et al. EAE/ASE recommendations for image acquisition and display using three-dimensional echocardiography. J Am Soc Echocardiogr 2012;25:3–46.

51. Elgharably H, Ibrahim A, Rosinski B, et al. Right heart failure and patient selection for isolated tricuspid valve surgery. J Thorac Cardiovasc Surg 2021. https://doi.org/10.1016/j.jtcvs.2021.10.059.

52. Taramasso M, Alessandrini H, Latib A, et al. Outcomes After Current Transcatheter Tricuspid Valve Intervention: Mid-Term Results From the International TriValve Registry. JACC Cardiovasc Interv 2019;12:155–65.

53. Muraru D, Haugaa K, Donal E, et al. Right ventricular longitudinal strain in the clinical routine: a state-of-the-art review. Eur Heart J Cardiovasc Imaging 2022;23:898–912.

54. Addetia K, Miyoshi T, Citro R, et al. Two-Dimensional Echocardiographic Right Ventricular Size and Systolic Function Measurements Stratified by Sex, Age, and Ethnicity: Results of the World Alliance of Societies of Echocardiography Study. J Am Soc Echocardiogr 2021;34:1148–57.e1.

55. Namisaki H, Nabeshima Y, Kitano T, et al. Prognostic Value of the Right Ventricular Ejection Fraction, Assessed by Fully Automated Three-Dimensional Echocardiography: A Direct Comparison of Analyses Using Right Ventricular-Focused Views versus Apical Four-Chamber Views. J Am Soc Echocardiogr 2021;34:117–26.

56. Muraru D, Badano LP, Nagata Y, et al. Development and prognostic validation of partition values to grade right ventricular dysfunction severity using 3D echocardiography. Eur Heart J Cardiovasc Imaging 2020;21:10–21.

57. Prihadi EA, van der Bijl P, Dietz M, et al. Prognostic Implications of Right Ventricular Free Wall Longitudinal Strain in Patients With Significant Functional Tricuspid Regurgitation. Circ Cardiovasc Imaging 2019;12:e008666.

58. Kresoja KP, Rommel KP, Lücke C, et al. Right Ventricular Contraction Patterns in Patients Undergoing Transcatheter Tricuspid Valve Repair for Severe Tricuspid Regurgitation. JACC Cardiovasc Interv 2021;1551–61.

59. Orban M, Wolff S, Braun D, et al. Right Ventricular Function in Transcatheter Edge-to-Edge Tricuspid Valve Repair. J Am Coll Cardiol 2021;14:2477–9.

60. Bosch L, Lam CSP, Gong L, et al. Right ventricular dysfunction in left-sided heart failure with preserved versus reduced ejection fraction. Eur J Heart Fail 2017;19:1664–71.

61. Melenovsky V, Hwang SJ, Lin G, et al. Right heart dysfunction in heart failure with preserved ejection fraction. Eur Heart J 2014;35:3452–62.

62. Hsu S, Simpson CE, Houston BA, et al. Multi-Beat Right Ventricular-Arterial Coupling Predicts Clinical Worsening in Pulmonary Arterial Hypertension. J Am Heart Assoc 2020;9:e016031.

63. Vanderpool RR, Pinsky MR, Naeije R, et al. RV-pulmonary arterial coupling predicts outcome in patients referred for pulmonary hypertension. Heart 2015;101:37–43.

64. Eleid MF, Padang R, Pislaru SV, et al. Effect of Transcatheter Aortic Valve Replacement on Right Ventricular-Pulmonary Artery Coupling. JACC Cardiovasc Interv 2019;12:2145–54.

65. Fortuni F, Butcher SC, Dietz MF, et al. Right Ventricular-Pulmonary Arterial Coupling in Secondary Tricuspid Regurgitation. Am J Cardiol 2021;148:138–45.

66. Brener MI, Lurz P, Hausleiter J, et al. Right Ventricular-Pulmonary Arterial Coupling and Afterload Reserve in Patients Undergoing Transcatheter Tricuspid Valve Repair. J Am Coll Cardiol 2022;79:448–61.

67. Lurz P, Orban M, Besler C, et al. Clinical characteristics, diagnosis, and risk stratification of pulmonary hypertension in severe tricuspid regurgitation and implications for transcatheter tricuspid valve repair. Eur Heart J 2020;41:2785–95.

68. Hahn RT. Finding concordance in discord: the value of discordant invasive and echocardiographic pulmonary artery pressure measurements with severe tricuspid regurgitation. Eur Heart J 2020;41:2796–8.

69. Hahn RT, Abraham T, Adams MS, et al. Guidelines for performing a comprehensive transesophageal echocardiographic examination: recommendations from the American Society of Echocardiography and the Society of Cardiovascular Anesthesiologists. J Am Soc Echocardiogr 2013;26:921–64.

70. Hahn RT, Saric M, Faletra FF, et al. Recommended Standards for the Performance of Transesophageal Echocardiographic Screening for Structural Heart Intervention: From the American Society of Echocardiography. J Am Soc Echocardiogr 2022;35:1–76.

71. Hagemeyer D, Ali FM, Ong G, et al. The Role of Intracardiac Echocardiography in Percutaneous Tricuspid Intervention: A New ICE Age. Interv Cardiol Clin 2022;11:103–12.

72. Møller JE, De Backer O, Nuyens P, et al. Transesophageal and intracardiac echocardiography to guide transcatheter tricuspid valve repair with the TriClip™ system. Int J Cardiovasc Imaging 2022;38:609–11.

73. Curio J, Abulgasim K, Kasner M, et al. Intracardiac echocardiography to enable successful edge-to-edge transcatheter tricuspid valve repair in patients with insufficient TEE quality. Clin Hemorheol Microcirc 2020;76:199–210.

74. Wong I, Chui ASF, Wong CY, et al. Complimentary Role of ICE and TEE During Transcatheter Edge-to-Edge Tricuspid Valve Repair With TriClip G4. JACC Cardiovasc Interv 2022;15:562–3.

75. Davidson CJ, Abramson S, Smith RL, et al. Trans-catheter Tricuspid Repair With the Use of 4-Dimensional Intracardiac Echocardiography. JACC Cardiovasc Imaging 2022;15:533–8.

76. Hinzpeter R, Eberhard M, Burghard P, et al. Computed tomography in patients with tricuspid regurgitation prior to transcatheter valve repair: dynamic analysis of the annulus with an individually tailored contrast media protocol. EuroIntervention 2017;12:e1828–36.

77. Henneman MM, Schuijf JD, Jukema JW, et al. Assessment of global and regional left ventricular function and volumes with 64-slice MSCT: a comparison with 2D echocardiography. J Nucl Cardiol 2006; 13:480–7.

78. Greupner J, Zimmermann E, Grohmann A, et al. Head-to-head comparison of left ventricular function assessment with 64-row computed tomography, biplane left cineventriculography, and both 2- and 3-dimensional transthoracic echocardiography: comparison with magnetic resonance imaging as the reference standard. J Am Coll Cardiol 2012;59: 1897–907.

79. Yeh BM, Kurzman P, Foster E, et al. Clinical relevance of retrograde inferior vena cava or hepatic vein opacification during contrast-enhanced CT. AJR Am J Roentgenol 2004;183:1227–32.

80. Prihadi EA, Delgado V, Hahn RT, et al. Imaging Needs in Novel Transcatheter Tricuspid Valve Interventions. JACC Cardiovasc Imaging 2018;11: 736–54.

81. Koch JA, Poll LW, Godehardt E, et al. Right and left ventricular volume measurements in an animal heart model in vitro: first experiences with cardiac MRI at 1.0 T. Eur Radiol 2000;10:455–8.

82. Jauhiainen T, Jarvinen VM, Hekali PE, et al. MR gradient echo volumetric analysis of human cardiac casts: focus on the right ventricle. J Comput Assist Tomogr 1998;22:899–903.

83. Baker KB, Tkach JA, Nyenhuis JA, et al. Evaluation of specific absorption rate as a dosimeter of MRI-related implant heating. J Magn Reson Imaging 2004;20:315–20.

84. Olivieri LJ, Cross RR, O'Brien KE, et al. Optimized protocols for cardiac magnetic resonance imaging in patients with thoracic metallic implants. Pediatr Radiol 2015;45:1455–64.

85. Rashid S, Rapacchi S, Vaseghi M, et al. Improved late gadolinium enhancement MR imaging for patients with implanted cardiac devices. Radiology 2014;270:269–74.

86. Symons R, Zimmerman SL, Bluemke DA. CMR and CT of the Patient With Cardiac Devices: Safety, Efficacy, and Optimization Strategies. JACC Cardiovasc Imaging 2019;12:890–903.

87. Hahn RT, Asch F, Weissman NJ, et al. Impact of Tricuspid Regurgitation on Clinical Outcomes: The COAPT Trial. J Am Coll Cardiol 2020;76:1305–14.

88. Stassen J, Galloo X, Hirasawa K, et al. Tricuspid regurgitation after cardiac resynchronization therapy: evolution and prognostic significance. Europace 2022;24:1291–9.

89. Vahanian A, Beyersdorf F, Praz F, et al. 2021 ESC/EACTS Guidelines for the management of valvular heart disease. Eur Heart J 2022;43:561–632.

Mitral Regurgitation
Advanced Imaging Parameters and Changing Treatment Landscape

Thomas Maher, MD[a], Andrea Vegh, MD[a], Seth Uretsky, MD, FSCMR[b],*

KEYWORDS

- Cardiovascular magnetic resonance • Echocardiography • Mitral regurgitation

KEY POINTS

- Cardiovascular magnetic resonance (CMR) is an accurate and reproducible imaging modality to assess mitral regurgitation severity.
- In head-to-head studies of echocardiography and CMR, CMR was a superior predictor of postsurgical left ventricular remodeling and clinical outcomes.
- CMR should be considered when deciding a patient's appropriateness for mitral valve surgery.

INTRODUCTION

Mitral regurgitation is the most frequent valvular heart disease in the United States and the second most common form of valvular heart disease requiring surgery in Europe.[1] Mitral regurgitation results when there is retrograde systolic flow from the left ventricle into the left atrium. It affects approximately 10% of the population aged older than 75 years, and the number of patients with mitral regurgitation are expected to increase given the aging population.[2] When mitral regurgitation is detected early in the disease process, allowing for appropriate intervention, the life expectancy of the patient can be preserved. This necessitates the need for early and accurate detection.[1]

CAUSES

The mitral valve is a complex 3-dimensional structure consisting of 2 leaflets (anterior and posterior leaflet), chordae, and papillary muscles. The papillary muscles are anchored to the left ventricular myocardium making the geometry of the left ventricle important to the functioning of the mitral valve apparatus. The fundamental problem in mitral regurgitation is the reduction or loss of coaptation between the anterior and posterior mitral leaflets resulting in poor mitral competence during ventricular systole. In primary (or degenerative) mitral regurgitation, the cause is due to a malfunction of the mitral valve itself, such as a prolapsed or flail leaflet, which inhibits complete leaflet coaptation during systole. In secondary (or functional) mitral regurgitation, the cause is not directly due to the malfunction of the valve but rather is the result of both ischemic and nonischemic changes. An example of secondary mitral regurgitation is dilatation of the mitral annulus secondary to dilated cardiomyopathy resulting in incomplete coaptation of the leaflets. In the Society of Thoracic Surgeons (STS) database, approximately 61% of mitral regurgitation requiring surgery is due to primary myxomatous disease with rheumatic disease (22.5%), ischemic disease (1.3%), endocarditis (5.1%), and nonischemic cardiomyopathies (2.9%) account for the rest.[3]

CURRENT THERAPIES

The therapies for mitral regurgitation depend on the etiology of the lesion. For patients with secondary mitral regurgitation due to dilated cardiomyopathy or ischemic disease, the first step is to treat the

[a] Department of Medicine, Morristown Medical Center, Morristown, NJ, USA; [b] Department of Cardiovascular Medicine, Gagnon Cardiovascular Institute, Morristown Medical Center/Atlantic Health System, 100 Madison Avenue, Morristown, NJ 07960, USA
* Corresponding author.
E-mail address: seth.uretsky@atlantichealth.org

Heart Failure Clin 19 (2023) 525–530
https://doi.org/10.1016/j.hfc.2023.05.001
1551-7136/23/© 2023 Elsevier Inc. All rights reserved.

underlying disease, which is done primarily with medical therapy and revascularization procedures for ischemic cause. For patients with primary mitral regurgitation, the therapeutic effect of medical therapy is limited and mitral valve surgery to repair or replace the valve is the mainstay of treatment. Mitral valve surgery, however, is not without risks, particularly in patients with comorbidities making them poor surgical candidates.[3,4] For patients at high risk for mitral valve surgery, minimally invasive procedures are actively being developed and studied. The MitraClip is the most widely used minimally invasive device but other devices are currently being studied.[5] Other devices include the Pascal Mitral Repair System, which is designed to approximate the mitral valve leaflets, and the Carillon mitral contour system, which improves leaflet coaptation by implanting into the coronary sinus and the great cardiac vein by applying tension along the posterior mitral annulus.[5] The success of transcatheter aortic valve replacement (TAVR) has also created a growing interest in the use of transcatheter mitral valve replacement devices including the Tendyne, the Intrepid, and the Sapien M3 valves.[5]

IMAGING

The timing for mitral valve intervention is guided by the American College of Cardiology/American Heart Association (ACC/AHA) recommendation for valvular heart disease.[6] The current recommendations focus on the severity of the mitral regurgitation as well as the presence or absence of symptoms. Although most experts agree that symptomatic patients with severe mitral regurgitation should be considered for mitral valve surgery, recommendations in asymptomatic patients remain controversial.[7,8]

The most common imaging modality used to assess the severity of mitral regurgitation is echocardiography. Echocardiography can be used to assess the severity of mitral regurgitation as well as the hemodynamic effects of the mitral regurgitant volume on the left ventricle and left atrium. As per the American Society of Echocardiography (ASE) guidelines, there are several parameters to qualify and quantify mitral regurgitation using echocardiography, including semiquantitative and quantitative parameters.[9] These parameters include the assessment of mitral valve morphology, left atrial and ventricular size, and semiquantitative and quantitative parameters. Semiquantitative and quantitative echocardiographic parameters include color flow jet area, continuous wave Doppler jet shape/density, pulmonary vein flow reversal, vena contracta, mitral inflow, proximal isovelocity surface area-based (PISA) regurgitant volume and effective regurgitant orifice area, and pulsed Doppler-based volumetric regurgitant volume and effective regurgitant orifice area.[9] Multiple parameters exist due to the lack of a single accurate and reproducible parameter as highlighted by Biner and colleagues and Thomas and colleagues.[10,11] The lack of a single reproducible echocardiographic parameter led to the use of the ASE-endorsed integrative method.[12] The integrative method focused on integrating multiple echocardiographic parameters, with particular emphasis on quantitative parameters, to assess the severity of mitral regurgitation. There are 2 major drawbacks to this method. First, it is unclear how the integration of parameters that lack reproducibility and lack accuracy can accurately diagnose the severity of mitral regurgitation. Second, studies have shown that there is significant discordance among the echocardiographic parameters in patients with mitral regurgitation,[10,13] yet the ASE guidelines did not guide echocardiographers as to how to weight each individual parameter. To better guide echocardiographers, the latest ASE guidelines suggest the use of an algorithm, which highlights parameters that are indicative of definitely mild and definitely severe mitral regurgitation.[9] However, even when using the ASE algorithm, echocardiographic parameters remain discordant in patients particularly in those with more severe mitral regurgitation. Uretsky and colleagues reported discordance in echocardiographic parameters in 92% of patients designated as definitely severe by the ASE algorithm and in 100% of patients with graded III/IV severe mitral regurgitation (MR) by the ASE algorithm.[13] This finding highlights the difficulty for echocardiographers in determining which patients have severe MR.

Recent studies have highlighted the accuracy of cardiovascular magnetic resonance (CMR) to quantify the severity of mitral regurgitation.[14–17] CMR quantification of mitral regurgitation uses the strengths of the CMR technique, namely quantifying the structure and function of the left and right ventricles and quantifying blood flow using phase contrast imaging[18] (Fig. 1). CMR has been recognized as the gold standard method to noninvasively quantify left and right ventricular volumes, ejection fractions, and stroke volumes. Phase contrast imaging is used to quantify blood flow in the ascending aorta and the pulmonary artery, which can be used to establish forward flow. Quantifying left ventricular volume is important because the primary adaptation of the left ventricle to mitral regurgitation is dilatation.[19] Studies have shown that mitral regurgitation, quantified using CMR, correlates well with the degree of left ventricular dilatation presurgery and

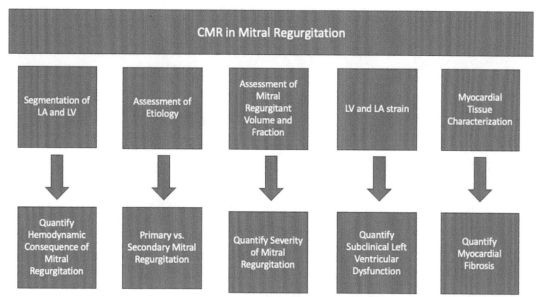

Fig. 1. CMR assessment of patients with mitral regurgitation. CMR can quantify the severity of valvular heart disease, determine the cause of MR, assess the hemodynamic effect on cardiac chambers, and assess myocardial fibrosis. CMR, Cardiovascular magnetic resonance.

remodeling postsurgery.[16,17,19] In addition, the left atrium dilates in patients with mitral regurgitation, and this also is an important indicator of the severity of mitral regurgitation. In patients with lone mitral regurgitation and no other valvular heart disease mitral regurgitation can be calculated as follows:

Mitral regurgitant volume = left ventricular stroke volume (LVSV) – forward flow.

Mitral regurgitant fraction = mitral regurgitant volume/LVSV.

Forward flow can be determined using ascending aorta phase contrast (AoPC), proximal pulmonary artery phase contrast (PAPC), right ventricular stroke volume (RVSV), or an average of all 3 (**Figs. 2** and **3**). Measuring forward flow using 3 different methods allows the interpreter to ensure that the data is consistent. *This method has been shown to have low interobserver variability and to be highly reproducible.*[17,19,20] Ideally, a CMR laboratory should measure all 4 data points (LVSV, RVSV, AoPC, and PAPC) on all patients undergoing CMR. In patients with no valvular heart disease or congenital heart disease, all 4 measurements should be equal to each other. This allows the CMR laboratory to ensure that the data acquisition and interpretation are accurate and can be trusted in patients with valvular heart disease and/or congenital heart disease. In patients with mitral and aortic regurgitation, aortic regurgitation can be measured directly using the diastolic flow on the AoPC, and the mitral regurgitation is calculated as follows:

Mitral regurgitant volume = LVSV – (forward flow + aortic regurgitation).

Studies have compared CMR and echocardiography in the quantification of mitral regurgitation.[14–17,21–23] These studies have shown significant discordance between CMR and echocardiography, particularly in patients with severe mitral regurgitation who are considered for referral for surgery. Of particular concern is the tendency for echocardiography to diagnose severe mitral regurgitation often in patients with nonsevere mitral regurgitation by CMR. Studies have compared individual echocardiographic parameters to CMR and have found that none of the echocardiographic parameters accurately diagnosed mitral regurgitation.[24,25] To date, there have been 4 studies comparing CMR and echocardiography with outcomes.[14–17] Two studies have compared CMR and echocardiography in patients undergoing surgery and found that mitral regurgitant volume quantified using CMR predicted the postsurgical remodeling of the left ventricle, and mitral regurgitant volume by echocardiography did not *predict the postsurgical remodeling of the left ventricle.*[16,17] In addition, mitral regurgitation determined using the ASE algorithm did not predict postsurgical remodeling of the left ventricle.[16] Of note, in both these studies, two-thirds of patients with severe mitral regurgitation by echocardiography had nonsevere mitral regurgitation by CMR.[16,17] Two studies have compared CMR and echocardiography in predicting clinical outcomes.[14,15] Both

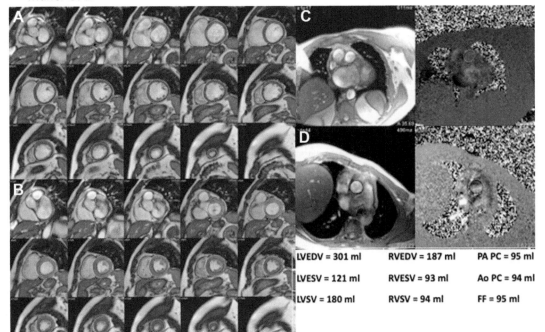

LVEDV = 301 ml	RVEDV = 187 ml	PA PC = 95 ml
LVESV = 121 ml	RVESV = 93 ml	Ao PC = 94 ml
LVSV = 180 ml	RVSV = 94 ml	FF = 95 ml

Fig. 2. Quantification of mitral regurgitation using CMR. Segmentation of (*A*) end-diastolic and (*B*) end-systolic volume of the left and right ventricles quantifies left and right stroke volumes. (*C*) PA PC and (*D*) AoPC quantifies flow in these vessels. Forward flow can be quantified using either RVSV, PA PC, AoPC, or an average of all of them. AoPC, ascending aorta phase contrast; FF, forward flow; LVEDV, left ventricular end-diastolic volume; LV ESV, left ventricular end-systolic volume; LVSV, left ventricular stroke volume; MR, mitral regurgitation; PA PC, pulmonary artery phase contrast; RVSV, right ventricular stroke volume.

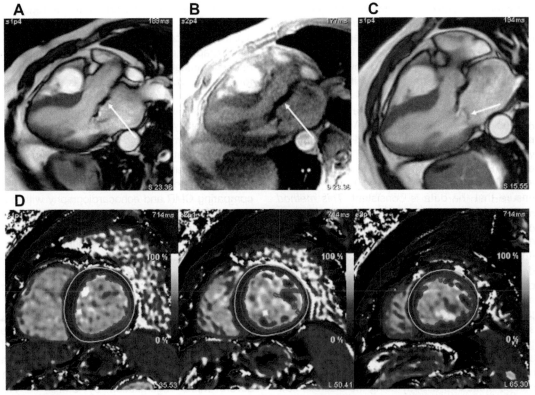

Fig. 3. (*A*) SSFP and (*B*) FSPGR 3 chamber view showing anteriorly directed mitral regurgitation (*arrows*). (*C*) SSFP off axis 3-chamber view showing posterior flail leaflet (*arrow*). (*D*) T1 mapping based extracellular volume of a basal, mid, and apical short axis view. Global ECV = 22%, which is consistent of the absence of diffuse myocardial fibrosis. FSPGR, Fast spoiled gradient echo; SSFP, steady state free precession.

studies found that mitral regurgitation by CMR predicted clinical outcomes while echocardiography did not. These findings are sobering when considering that echocardiography is used to decide when patients are referred for surgery and more often diagnoses severe MR. Based on these studies, there is concern that patients with nonsevere mitral regurgitation are being referred for mitral valve surgery.

CMR is also capable of performing tissue characterization of the left ventricular myocardium. T1 mapping techniques have been validated in detecting diffuse interstitial fibrosis as measured by extracellular volume (ECV).[26,27] Edwards and colleagues showed that asymptomatic patients with moderate-to-severe mitral regurgitation had signs of myocardial fibrosis associated with reduced myocardial deformation and reduced exercise tolerance.[26] The concern is that there are asymptomatic patients that may benefit from early intervention to help reduce irreversible changes that are currently not being recommended for surgery. Additional research by Kitkungvan and colleagues showed that elevated ECV was independently associated with symptoms related to mitral regurgitation.[27] There needs to be more research to determine ECV thresholds but the hope is that ECV can be used by clinicians to detect subclinical changes before severe reductions in left ventricular function. This could result in more patients being recommended for surgery and being better surgical candidates.

SUMMARY

Although echocardiography is often the first test performed in patients with valvular heart disease, recent studies have shown that CMR is a more accurate tool to quantify the severity of valvular heart disease. In addition, CMR is the gold standard for noninvasive evaluation of cardiac chamber structure and function and, thus, the best modality to assess the hemodynamic effect valve disease has on the heart. Exciting advancements in the field of CMR tissue characterization allows quantification of the fibrotic process that may occur due to volume and/or pressure overload on the left ventricle because of valvular heart disease.

CLINICS CARE POINT

- In patients being considered for surgery for mitral regurgitation, consider CMR to quantify severity of mitral regurgitation.

DISCLOSURE

The authors have nothing to disclose.

REFERENCES

1. Enriquez-Sarano M, Akins CW, Vahanian A. Mitral regurgitation. Lancet 2009;373:1382–94.
2. Grayburn PA, Weissman NJ, Zamorano JL. Quantitation of mitral regurgitation. Circulation 2012;126: 2005–17.
3. Gammie JS, Chikwe J, Badhwar V, et al. Isolated Mitral valve surgery: the society of thoracic surgeons adult cardiac surgery database analysis. Ann Thorac Surg 2018;106:716–27.
4. Suri RM, Vanoverschelde JL, Grigioni F, et al. Association between early surgical intervention vs watchful waiting and outcomes for mitral regurgitation due to flail mitral valve leaflets. JAMA 2013;310:609–16.
5. Lipiecki J, Kuzemczak M, Siminiak T. Transcatheter treatment of functional mitral valve regurgitation. Trends Cardiovasc Med 2021;31:487–94.
6. Writing Committee M, Otto CM, Nishimura RA, et al. 2020 ACC/AHA guideline for the management of patients with valvular heart disease: a report of the American college of cardiology/american heart association joint committee on clinical practice guidelines. J Am Coll Cardiol 2021;77:e25–197.
7. Enriquez-Sarano M, Sundt TM 3rd. Early surgery is recommended for mitral regurgitation. Circulation 2010;121:804–11 [discussion: 812].
8. Gillam LD, Schwartz A. Primum non nocere: the case for watchful waiting in asymptomatic "severe" degenerative mitral regurgitation. Circulation 2010; 121:813–21 [discussion: 821].
9. Zoghbi WA, Adams D, Bonow RO, et al. Recommendations for noninvasive evaluation of native valvular regurgitation: a report from the American society of echocardiography developed in collaboration with the society for cardiovascular magnetic resonance. J Am Soc Echocardiogr 2017;30:303–71.
10. Biner S, Rafique A, Rafii F, et al. Reproducibility of proximal isovelocity surface area, vena contracta, and regurgitant jet area for assessment of mitral regurgitation severity. JACC Cardiovasc Imaging 2010;3:235–43.
11. Thomas N, Unsworth B, Ferenczi EA, et al. Intraobserver variability in grading severity of repeated identical cases of mitral regurgitation. Am Heart J 2008;156:1089–94.
12. Zoghbi WA, Enriquez-Sarano M, Foster E, et al. Recommendations for evaluation of the severity of native valvular regurgitation with two-dimensional and Doppler echocardiography. J Am Soc Echocardiogr 2003;16:777–802.
13. Uretsky S, Aldaia L, Marcoff L, et al. Concordance and discordance of echocardiographic parameters

recommended for assessing the severity of mitral regurgitation. Circ Cardiovasc Imaging 2020;13:e010278.

14. Myerson SG, d'Arcy J, Christiansen JP, et al. Determination of clinical outcome in mitral regurgitation with cardiovascular magnetic resonance quantitation. Circulation 2016;133:2287–96.

15. Penicka M, Vecera J, Mirica DC, et al. Prognostic implications of magnetic resonance-derived quantification in asymptomatic patients with organic mitral regurgitation: comparison with doppler echocardiography-derived integrative approach. Circulation 2018;137:1349–60.

16. Uretsky S, Animashaun IB, Sakul S, et al. American society of echocardiography algorithm for degenerative mitral regurgitation: comparison with CMR. JACC Cardiovasc Imaging 2022;15:747–60.

17. Uretsky S, Gillam L, Lang R, et al. Discordance between echocardiography and MRI in the assessment of mitral regurgitation severity: a prospective multicenter trial. J Am Coll Cardiol 2015;65:1078–88.

18. Uretsky S, Argulian E, Narula J, et al. Use of cardiac magnetic resonance imaging in assessing mitral regurgitation: current evidence. J Am Coll Cardiol 2018;71:547–63.

19. Uretsky S, Supariwala A, Nidadovolu P, et al. Quantification of left ventricular remodeling in response to isolated aortic or mitral regurgitation. J Cardiovasc Magn Reson 2010;12:32.

20. Cawley PJ, Hamilton-Craig C, Owens DS, et al. Prospective comparison of valve regurgitation quantitation by cardiac magnetic resonance imaging and transthoracic echocardiography. Circ Cardiovasc Imaging 2013;6:48–57.

21. Lopez-Mattei JC, Ibrahim H, Shaikh KA, et al. Comparative assessment of mitral regurgitation severity by transthoracic echocardiography and cardiac magnetic resonance using an integrative and quantitative approach. Am J Cardiol 2016;117:264–70.

22. Sachdev V, Hannoush H, Sidenko S, et al. Are echocardiography and CMR really discordant in mitral regurgitation? JACC Cardiovasc Imaging 2017;10(7):823–4.

23. Altes A, Levy F, Iacuzio L, et al. Comparison of mitral regurgitant volume assessment between proximal flow convergence and volumetric methods in patients with significant primary mitral regurgitation: an echocardiographic and cardiac magnetic resonance imaging study. J Am Soc Echocardiogr 2022;35:671–81.

24. Uretsky S, Argulian E, Supariwala A, et al. A Comparative assessment of echocardiographic parameters for determining primary mitral regurgitation severity using magnetic resonance imaging as a reference standard. J Am Soc Echocardiogr 2018;31:992–9.

25. Uretsky S, Morales DCV, Aldaia L, et al. Characterization of primary mitral regurgitation with flail leaflet and/or wall-impinging flow. J Am Coll Cardiol 2021;78:2537–46.

26. Edwards NC, Moody WE, Yuan M, et al. Quantification of left ventricular interstitial fibrosis in asymptomatic chronic primary degenerative mitral regurgitation. Circ Cardiovasc Imaging 2014;7:946–53.

27. Kitkungvan D, Yang EY, El Tallawi KC, et al. Prognostic implications of diffuse interstitial fibrosis in asymptomatic primary mitral regurgitation. Circulation 2019;140:2122–4.

Emerging Roles for Artificial Intelligence in Heart Failure Imaging

Andrew J. Bradley, MD*, Malik Ghawanmeh, MD, Ashley M. Govi, MD,
Pedro Covas, MD, Gurusher Panjrath, MD, Andrew D. Choi, MD

KEYWORDS

- Heart failure • Artificial intelligence • Cardiac imaging • Cardiomyopathy • Machine learning

KEY POINTS

- Artificial intelligence (AI) applications are expanding in cardiac imaging.
- AI research has shown promise in workflow optimization, disease diagnosis, and integration of clinical and imaging data to predict patient outcomes.
- This review discusses areas of current research and potential clinical applications in AI as applied to heart failure cardiac imaging.

INTRODUCTION

Heart failure is a global pandemic; in the United States alone from 2015 to 2018 about 6 million Americans over the age of 20 had heart failure.[1] Prevalence of heart failure is projected to increase by 46% from 2012 to 2030, affecting greater than 8 million adult individuals. The total percentage of the population with HF is projected to rise from 2.4% in 2012 to 3.0% in 2030.[2] Because heart failure pathophysiology is related to both structural and functional abnormalities, accurately diagnosing and managing heart failure is often challenging.[3] Proper diagnosis and management of heart failure require the integration of a large variety of information, including clinical signs and symptoms, laboratory information, invasive hemodynamics, coronary physiologic data, and imaging.

Artificial intelligence (AI) has the potential to transform cardiovascular diagnosis and treatment by interpreting and finding meaning in large data sets more efficiently and effectively than human brains.[4] By interpreting images rapidly and consistently, AI has many possible benefits—time savings, reduced interobserver variability, and avoidance of errors due to fatigue or distraction. Additionally, it can integrate imaging and non-imaging data to guide diagnosis and management in the clinic. In this review article, we introduce the basic AI lexicon for the practicing clinician and discuss the emerging role of AI in multimodality heart failure imaging.

BASIC TERMINOLOGY OF ARTIFICIAL INTELLIGENCE

AI is the use of computer systems to perform complex tasks that require human intelligence.[5] Conceptually, the simplest AI is rule-based wherein inputs are processed according to human-defined rules (**Fig. 1**). By contrast, machine learning (ML) is a process in which computers learn patterns from data. With ML, the rules are not made by humans but instead are learned by the computer based on training data and experience.[6] ML is itself an umbrella term that includes a wide variety of algorithms that can learn and improve with experience.[7] Subdivisions of ML include supervised and unsupervised learning. Supervised learning identifies

Division of Cardiology, Department of Medicine, The George Washington University School of Medicine and Health Sciences, Washington, DC, USA
* Corresponding author. Division of Cardiology, The George Washington University School of Medicine, 2150 Pennsylvania Avenue Northwest Suite 4-417, Washington, DC.
E-mail address: abradley@mfa.gwu.edu
Twitter: @PanjrathG (G.P.); @AChoiHeart (A.D.C.)

Heart Failure Clin 19 (2023) 531–543
https://doi.org/10.1016/j.hfc.2023.03.005
1551-7136/23/

AI, Machine Learning and Deep Learning

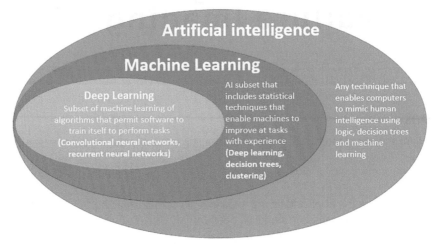

Artificial intelligence

Machine Learning

Deep Learning
Subset of machine learning of algorithms that permit software to train itself to perform tasks (Convolutional neural networks, recurrent neural networks)

AI subset that includes statistical techniques that enable machines to improve at tasks with experience (Deep learning, decision trees, clustering)

Any technique that enables computers to mimic human intelligence using logic, decision trees and machine learning

Fig. 1. A general hierarchy of the AI methods discussed in this article.

patterns in large data sets that are typically labeled by humans.[8] It is typically used to develop models that will predict or classify future events or to find the most relevant variables to the outcome.[9] In contrast, unsupervised learning analyzes large amounts of unlabeled data to identify hidden patterns and new relationships within the data.[10] Unsupervised learning seeks to identify novel disease mechanisms, genotypes, or phenotypes from hidden patterns present in data, without feedback from humans.[11] Deep learning (DL) is a particular branch of ML that uses multi-layered neural networks to find patterns in extensive data sets.[12] Modeled after human neurobiology, computer neural networks analyze complex patterns of inputs to produce a single output.[8] Neural networks learn through experience. Using neural networks, DL allows algorithms to respond correctly to completely new data using the previously added data sets. DL can produce actionable clinical information from diverse data sets and has numerous emerging applications in medicine and cardiology.[12]

ECHOCARDIOGRAPHY

Echocardiography offers simple, reliable, accessible evaluation of cardiac morphology and function through ultrasound imaging. It is often included in the initial evaluation of an individual with suspected heart failure. However, the interpretation of a complex echocardiogram can be time-consuming. AI software may save time by performing a preliminary analysis of echocardiographic images, for example, by quickly determining parameters of left ventricular ejection

fraction or longitudinal strain.[13] Emerging AI applications include the assessment of diastolic function, cardiomyopathy classification, and valvular lesions.

Left Ventricular Ejection Fraction and Cardiomyopathy Assessment

Global systolic function is one of the most important parameters assessed in echocardiography. Recent approaches have sought to train AI to mimic both the visual estimate and automate the quantification of ejection fraction. Integration of multi-faceted left ventricular (LV) function beyond ejection fraction to include global longitudinal strain is highly attractive. Video-based DL algorithms can estimate the left ventricular ejection fraction (LVEF) with less variability than human experts and can track changes in LVEF over time.[14,15]

Automated echocardiogram interpretation extends beyond routine echocardiographic parameters such as chambers structure and function to identify cardiomyopathies of distinct etiologies: hypertrophic cardiomyopathy (HCM), cardiac amyloidosis, pulmonary arterial hypertension (PAH), and chemotherapy-induced cardiomyopathy. Echocardiographic features associated with these cardiomyopathies can be subtle and easily missed. AI is being evaluated to detect these features through training on a large volume of echocardiographic images and clinical data.[16]

Zhang and colleagues explored the ability of convolutional neural networks (CNN) to provide fully automated evaluation of echocardiographic images. CNNs were trained in view classification, chamber segmentation, and recognition of three diseases: HCM, cardiac amyloid, and PAH. The reliability of segmentation was evaluated by using the results to calculate chamber volumes and metrics such as left atrial volume, LVEF, and global longitudinal strain (GLS). LVEF accuracy was evaluated on 6407 echocardiograms with an average absolute error of 6%. Automated GLS compared with 418 manual GLS calculations had an average absolute error of 1.4%. Left atrial volume in 4800 studies was accurate to within 9% in half of the echocardiograms. From a disease diagnosis standpoint, AI was able to detect HCM (495 case echocardiograms, 2244 control echocardiograms) with an area under the receiving operating characteristic curve (AUC) of 0.93 (95% CI, 0.91–0.94). Similarly, the model was able to detect cardiac amyloid (179 case echocardiograms, 804 control echocardiograms) with an AUC of 0.87 (95% CI, 0.83–0.91). Finally, using the right ventricular structure and function abnormalities, the model was able to predict PAH (584 case echocardiograms, 2487 control echocardiograms) with an AUC of 0.85 (95% CI, 0.83–0.86).[16]

Diastolic Function Assessment

Echocardiography is essential for diastolic function assessment, but complex in incorporating multiple criteria. The American Society of Echocardiography and European Association of Cardiovascular Imaging (ASE/EACVI) guidelines are widely adopted for diastolic function assessment, using two algorithms to screen for and grade diastolic dysfunction.[17] ML may help to decrease indeterminate diastolic function assessment, predict and improve long-term outcomes, and personalize prognosis prediction, automated staging, and disease progression monitoring in these patients.[18,19]

Pandey and colleagues investigated a Deep Neural Network (DeepNN) model for diastolic dysfunction evaluation that used multiple key echocardiographic parameters.[20] This model was compared against the ASE diastolic dysfunction guidelines for its ability to predict elevated LV filling pressures. It was also applied to patients in the TOPCAT, RELAX-HF, and NEAT-HFpEF trials to evaluate its correlation with clinically meaningful outcomes. The DeepNN model was better than the ASE guidelines at predicting elevated LV filling pressure in a reference group of patients undergoing both echocardiography and invasive hemodynamic measurement (AUC 0.88 vs 0.67). Additionally, patients judged to be high risk by the DeepNN model had lower survival rates,

more abnormal cardiac biomarkers, and lower exercise tolerance in the clinical trial populations. Importantly, the DeepNN was able to reduce the number of patients classified by guidelines as having an indeterminate diastolic function and explicitly stratified them as high or low risk.

Right Ventricular Function Assessment

The right ventricle (RV) has a complex pyramidal shape making functional and structural assessment challenging and time-consuming. ML has been applied to the analysis of RV function on both 2D and 3D echocardiography using cardiac MRI (CMR) as the reference standard. In a feasibility study where CMR-derived RV ejection fraction of less than 50% defined patients with RV dysfunction, Beecy and colleagues demonstrated that an ML algorithm could track the tricuspid annulus and identify RV dysfunction similarly to conventional parameters (AUC for ML parameters 0.69–0.75; AUC for TAPSE 0.80).[21] Genovese and colleagues tested an ML algorithm for RV size and function quantification on 3D echocardiography with excellent reliability (eg, right ventricular ejection fraction [RVEF] bias $-3.3\% \pm 5.2\%$). In 32% of patients, the software could contour the RV automatically in approximately 15 seconds while the remainder required contour editing by a human reader, adding approximately 114 seconds to the analysis.[22]

Valvular Heart Diseases Assessment

Echocardiographic assessment is essential in diagnosing valvular heart diseases (VHD). Using image recognition and integrating echocardiographic and clinical data, AI has the potential to phenotype patients and predict worse outcomes promoting precision medicine and individualized care for VHD patients.[23] AI has been studied for sizing of transcatheter aortic valve replacement (TAVR) and predicting survival after TAVR.[24,25] CNN were applied by Zhang and colleagues to Doppler echocardiography images and could accurately identify the severity of MR per the ASE 2017 guidelines.[26] 3D echocardiography is also widely used to diagnose MR and guide interventional planning. Chen and colleagues compared an AI segmentation model with clinical software performance in measuring the mitral valve annular parameters. The automatic segmentation model provided comparable results with precision: dice similarity coefficient of 0.877 $\pm$ 0.027 and an average surface distance of 0.925 $\pm$ 0.392 mm.[27] Kagiyama and colleagues confirmed that 3D automated mitral valve quantification provides faster analysis time than manual tracing (260 ± 65 vs 381 ± 68 seconds) with similar accuracy.[28] Additionally, AI may potentially be used to simulate, predict the chances of success, and plan transcatheter edge-to-edge repair (Mitra-Clip procedure).[29]

NUCLEAR IMAGING AND CARDIAC COMPUTED TOMOGRAPHY TO ASSESS ISCHEMIC CARDIOMYOPATHY

Defining the etiology of cardiomyopathy requires an understanding of the patient's coronary physiology; nuclear imaging, particularly single photon emission computed tomography (SPECT) is the prototypical modality used to evaluate myocardial perfusion. Cardiac computed tomography (CT) provides highly accurate and rapid visualization of the coronary arteries and aids in the exclusion of obstructive coronary artery disease and the identification of ischemic cardiomyopathy.[30]

Machine Learning Analysis of Nuclear Studies

Arsanjani and colleagues explored, in two studies, the application of ML in the evaluation of nuclear perfusion imaging using invasive coronary angiography as the reference standard for hemodynamically significant coronary stenosis. The outcomes were the accurate detection of coronary artery disease and early (ie, within 90 days after perfusion imaging) revascularization. Automatically-calculated perfusion imaging parameters such as total perfusion deficit and transient ischemic dilation were combined with clinical features such as patient sex and post-stress electrocardiogram (ECG) likelihood of coronary artery disease as inputs into the ML algorithm. Compared with expert readers who had access to clinical data, ML demonstrated similar accuracy (87.3%), sensitivity (78.9%), and specificity (92.1%) for the detection of coronary artery disease (CAD).[31] ML was also comparable to expert interpretation at predicting the need for early revascularization with an AUC of 0.81.[32]

The ability of a DL algorithm to analyze SPECT polar maps in concert with certain clinical variables (age, sex, LV end-systolic and diastolic volumes) and identify obstructive coronary disease was evaluated by Otaki and colleagues. Trained on 3578 patients who underwent both SPECT and invasive angiography (where left main stenosis ≥50% or any other main vessel ≥70% defined obstructive disease), the DL algorithm was then validated on a separate data set of 555 patients, achieving an AUC of 0.80 versus 0.65 by human readers. Importantly, this software produces results in under 12 seconds and includes attention maps to highlight for a human reader the segments of the polar map contributing most to its predictions.[33]

Machine Learning Determination of Computed Tomography-Fractional Flow Reserve and Obstructive CAD by Cardiac Computed Tomography

Invasive fractional flow reserve (FFR) obtained during coronary angiography is the reference standard for assessing the hemodynamic significance of coronary artery stenoses.[34] However, advancements in computational flow dynamics (CFD) and imaging-based modeling have allowed for FFR to be computed from CT angiography (CTA) images, yielding CT-FFR.[35] This non-invasive calculation of FFR requires accurate anatomic segmentation and modeling of vascular resistance and compliance. As an alternative to the traditional CFD-calculated CT-FFR, Itu and colleagues developed an ML-based model to predict FFR by training the algorithm on 12,000 synthetic coronary trees for which CFD-based CT-FFR had been calculated.[36] Their model reduced execution time by more than 80 times and the correlation between their ML model and conventional physics-based models was 0.9994 (P <.001). Itu's model, initially validated against invasive CFD-based CT-FFR and invasive FFR in 87 patients, was further validated by Coenen and colleagues who compared its diagnostic performance against CFD-based CT-FFR, visual CTA analysis, and invasive FFR in a multi-center cohort of 351 patients.[37] Correlation between ML-based and CFD-based CT-FFR was excellent (R = 0.997). Using invasive FFR as the reference standard, ML-based CT-FRR had improved per-patient accuracy (71% by visual CTA analysis vs 85% by ML-based CT-FRR). Importantly, ML-based CT-FFR correctly identified 73% of false-positive visual CTA results.

The CT Evaluation by Artificial Intelligence for Atherosclerosis, Stenosis and Vascular Morphology (CLARIFY) multi-center study by Choi and colleagues compared AI using a series of CNN to level 3 (L3) readers in detecting coronary artery stenosis on CCTA. The AI analysis showed 99.7% accuracy in detecting greater than 70% stenosis and 94.8% accuracy in detecting greater than 50% stenosis.[38] A subsequent analysis by Griffin and colleagues evaluated a multi-center cohort of patients undergoing core-lab quantitative invasive angiography (QCA) and found that AI-based direct image for quantitative CT (AI-QCT) had high diagnostic accuracy when compared with QCA in detecting greater than 50% stenosis (AUC 0.88) and greater than 70% stenosis (AUC 0.92). In addition, AI-QCT provided accuracy (AUC 0.9) that is similar to QCA (AUC

0.9) against a standard of FFR less than 0.8.[38,39] AI-QCT by Lipkin and colleagues also found AI-QCT to have superior diagnosic performance compared to myocardial perfusion imaging (MPI). Using cutoffs of stenosis $\geq$ 50% or $\geq$70% by QCA, AI-QCT achieved an AUC of 0.88 and 0.92 whereas the AUC of MPI was 0.66 and 0.81, respectively. Similarly, using a standard of FFR less than 0.8, AI-QCT had an AUC of 0.90 vs 0.71 for MPI.[40]

CARDIAC MRI

Cardiac MRI (CMR) provides excellent tissue characterization for the evaluation of cardiomyopathies as well as accurate evaluation of ventricular function.[41–44] There are multiple aspects of CMR from image segmentation to outcome prediction that may benefit from AI.

Automated Segmentation

Segmentation, the process of identifying the myocardial borders, is a fundamental task in CMR analysis.[45] A normally tedious process, efforts to use AI to aid in segmentation have led to studies that have shown performances similar to human readers. In a study by Bai, automated chamber size quantifications yielded excellent agreement compared with human readers.[46] CNNs for fully automated LVEF calculation in a multi-vendor and multi-center study yielded a high correlation between the different vendors and centers.[47] ML algorithms for LVEF calculation were directly compared with human readers in a study by Davies.[48] The authors created a DL algorithm trained on 1923 scans. They found that the machine quantification was faster than human readers (20 seconds vs 13 minutes) with few errors that occurred on rare pathologies not encountered in training. Additionally, machine learning was more precise than human readers with rescan coefficients of variation for LVEF of 6.0% for humans and 4.2% in ML. A recent study by Chauhan and colleagues sought to compare the ability of ML (specifically a k-nearest neighbors algorithm) and DL to classify anatomic views on CMR. After being trained on approximately 60 cases, both ML and DL showed accuracy exceeding 0.98 but the accuracy dropped to under 0.85 when confronted with a population enriched for complex anatomy.[49]

The complex anatomy of the RV can cause variability in the estimation of the right ventricular function by CMR with human readers.[50–52] Despite these limitations, DL models have been developed to estimate the right ventricular function with similar reproducibility to human readers.[53] In a study by Wang and colleagues, 200 patients who completed a stress CMR had LVEF, LV mass

(LVM), and RVEF analyzed by DL algorithms and a clinician expert. The highest correlations between DL and clinician experts were for LVEF (r = 0.83–0.93) and LVM (r = 0.75–0.85). The correlation between DL and clinician for RVEF was lower (r = 0.59–0.68).[54] Following the results, the authors performed a subsequent study on the 100 patients with the largest discrepancies in RVEF. A second DL algorithm with an additional 10,161 images consisting of increased right ventricular pathology (eg, repaired Tetralogy of Fallot, PAH) was added to the cross-validation process. The new algorithm produced increased correlation for RVEF when compared with the original method (R = 0.87 vs R = 0.42).[55] The RVEF values were also categorized into $\leq$35%, 35% to 50%, and $\geq$50%. The updated algorithm showed increased accuracy for categorizing RV function when compared with the original (0.80 vs 0.53) with the lowest rates of accurate classifications in the 35% to 50% category.

Tissue Characterization

Tissue characterization may reasonably be considered the most valuable asset of CMR evaluating heart failure patients. The prototypical tissue characterization CMR sequence is late gadolinium enhancement (LGE) imaging. LGE imaging identifies myocardial fibrosis, whether non-ischemic or due to infarction, the pattern of which provides clues to the diagnosis; work has been done applying DL to the automatic quantification of scarring on LGE.[56] Additionally, there is considerable interest in identifying cardiomyopathies without the use of gadolinium contrast by using newer techniques such as T1 and T2 mapping which would reduce scan times and expand patient access. A recent study by Zhang and colleagues assessed the ability of CNN, using pre-contrast native T1 maps and cine images, to produce virtual native enhancement (VNE) images as an analog to traditional LGE images. A data set from the Hypertrophic Cardiomyopathy Registry comprising 1348 patients was used to train and test the model. Human experts scored the VNE highly for visuospatial agreement with LGE. Additionally, agreement of VNE with LGE for the extent of fibrosis (as a percentage of LVM) was high (r = 0.77–0.79 for hyperintense lesions, r = 0.70–0.76 for intermediate-intensity lesions).[57]

Outcomes

There is significant interest in predicting outcomes of patients with heart failure. Fahmy and colleagues trained an ML algorithm to consider CMR and clinical parameters to predict the composite outcome of death or cardiovascular hospitalization using a cohort of 229 patients with non-ischemic heart failure with reduced ejection fraction. This algorithm was then externally validated on a separate cohort of 214 patients, achieving an AUC of 0.69. Importantly, this model was designed to identify factors contributing to its predictions and highlighted markers of right ventricular dysfunction and remodeling as being of particular importance.[58]

Dawes and colleagues studied 256 patients with recently diagnosed PAH who underwent CMR, right heart catheterization, and a 6-minute walk test.[59] 3D cine recreations of the right ventricular function were used to estimate RVEF and right ventricular wall motion. Supervised ML was used to create risk prediction models based on the 3D wall motion to find areas predictive of survival. In a cohort with high mortality (36%) at 4 years, poor outcomes were predicted by a loss of effective contraction in the septum and free wall, coupled with reduced basal longitudinal motion. When hemodynamic data, biomarkers, and clinical information were added to 3D wall motion analysis, the survival prediction improved (AUC 0.73 vs 0.60; P <.001).

DISCUSSION

The possible roles of AI in the imaging of heart failure have been illustrated above and can be broadly divided into categories of (1) imaging lab workflow efficiency, (2) image-based diagnosis, and (3) prognostication. Additionally, AI may be designed to consider not only imaging data but also clinical information (**Fig. 2**, **Table 1**). For tasks like chamber quantification to simplify workflow or image-based diagnosis, AI accepts the actual images as input. For the category of clinical and imaging data integration, both measurements and data points from the imaging studies (whether automatically or manually generated) or the images themselves may be inputs to the model.

Management of heart failure requires a multidisciplinary team approach. From the standpoint of the individual clinician, the value of AI may vary depending on their clinical role (see **Fig. 2**). For example, a cardiac imager could use AI to carry out traditionally tedious tasks such as quantifying LVEF on echocardiogram or quantification of ventricular chamber volumes by CMR, freeing up time to focus on more nuanced aspects of image interpretation.[14,15,46] Good-quality VNE may eliminate

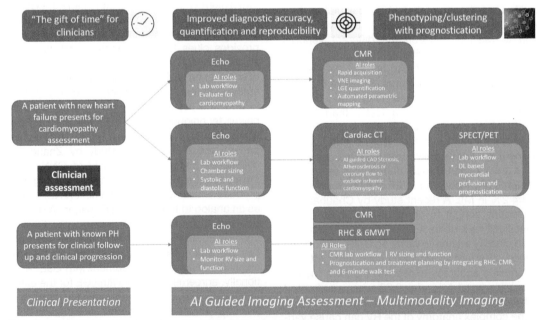

Fig. 2. Future paradigm of AI in heart failure assessment. The figure demonstrates the potential role of AI in two general hypothetical patient scenarios. In scenario 1, a patient presents with new heart failure for cardiomyopathy assessment. An initial echocardiogram may be rapidly assessed through acquisition and chamber quantification. After the initial assessment, a targeted approach (that avoids layered testing) may include assessment of cardiomyopathy through scar quantification or automation of parametric mapping. Ischemic cardiomyopathy assessment may use cardiac CT guided by AI or SPECT/PET imaging that uses DL for assessment of myocardial perfusion. In scenario 2, a patient with known PH may benefit from echo and CMR assessment. Prognostication and treatment planning may be guided by AI integration of the various clinical parameters.

Table 1
Summary of studies highlighting the role of artificial intelligence at different points of patient evaluation and management

Citation	Modality	Role for AI	Algorithm Type	Training or Derivation Cohort	Output	Ground Truth, Comparator And/or External Validation
Zhang et al,[16] 2018	Echo	Lab workflow Image diagnosis	DL	• 277 echoes with 791 images to train on view classification and segmentation • 495 HCM echoes with 2244 matched controls • 179 amyloid echoes with 804 matched controls • 584 PAH echoes with 2487 matched controls	• View classification, Chamber volumes, LVEF, GLS, diagnoses of HCM, amyloid, PAH	• >14,000 echoes used in total for testing • Human view classification • Human segmentations/tracings • Clinical diagnoses
Pandey et al,[20] 2021	Echo	Lab workflow Image diagnosis Prognostication	DL	• 1242 echoes	• High- or low-risk diastolic function	• Invasive hemodynamics (84 patients) • Clinical outcomes (512 patients in TOPCAT) • Biomarkers and 6-min walk (326 patients from RELAX-HF and NEAT-HFpEF)
Genovese et al,[22] 2019	Echo	Lab workflow	ML	• Large annotated data set (this article was on evaluation of a commercial product)	• Right ventricular volume from 3D echo • Time to perform measurements (including time to correct contours) reported in study	• Compared against CMR measurements of RV volumes obtained the same day (56 patients)
Arsanjani et al,[31] 2013	SPECT *plus clinical data*	Lab workflow Image diagnosis	LogitBoost	• 1181 SPECT studies	• Prediction of obstructive CAD	• Ground truth: invasive angiography • Compared against human readers
Otaki et al,[33] 2013	SPECT *plus clinical data*	Lab workflow Image diagnosis	DL	• 3578 SPECT studies with matching invasive angiography	• Presence of ischemia	• Ground truth: invasive angiography • Compared and validated against human reads in a separate cohort of 555 patients

(continued on next page)

Table 1
(continued)

Citation	Modality	Role for AI	Algorithm Type	Training or Derivation Cohort	Output	Ground Truth, Comparator And/or External Validation
Itu et al,[36] 2016 Coenen et al,[37] 2013	CCT	Lab workflow Image diagnosis	DL	• 12,000 synthetic coronary trees	• ML-derived CT-FFR	• Ground truth: invasive FFR • Itu validated in 87 patients against CFD-CT-FFR and invasive FFR • Coenen validated in 351 patients against CFD-CT-FFR, invasive FFR, and visual CTA interpretation
Choi et al,[38] 2021	CCT	Lab workflow Image diagnosis	DL	• Previously trained FDA-cleared algorithm	• Coronary segmentation, plaque quantification, lumen determination	• Ground truth: scan interpretation by three expert human readers • Data set comprised 232 patients
Davies et al,[48] 2022	CMR	Lab workflow	DL	• 1923 scans	• LV volume and EF • LVM	• Ground truth: human segmentation • Compared and validated against human reads in an additional 109 patients • Tested for generalizability in an external data set of 1277 patients
Wang,[54,55] 2022	CMR	Lab workflow	DL	• 200 scans initially • Additional ~1950 images enriched for RV pathology used for second study	• LVEF • LVM • RVEF	• Ground truth: human segmentation • Three commercial DL algorithms were compared against each other and to human segmentation in the initial study

Fahmy et al,[58] 2022	CMR *plus clinical data*	Prognostication	XGBoost	• 230 patients	• Risk of death or CV hospitalization • Identification of patient-specific risk factors driving the prediction	• Second study compared the original DL algorithm and an updated DL algorithm against human segmentation • Ground truth: clinical outcomes • Validated against a further 312 patients including 214 from a separate center
Dawes et al,[59] 2017	CMR *plus clinical data*	Prognostication	ML	• 256 patients undergoing CMR, right heart catheterization, and six-min walk test	• Prediction of survival	• Clinical outcomes
Zhang et al,[57] 2021	CMR	Lab workflow	DL	• 1348 patients (90% for training, 10% for validation)	• VNE imaging	• Ground truth: LGE imaging • Assessed by humans against LGE for visuospatial similarity • Extent of LGE (as % of LVM) quantified on VNE and correlated against LGE

the need for gadolinium contrast administration in CMR thus speeding acquisition, improving patient throughput, and ultimately increasing patient access to CMR.[57] When properly trained on large volumes of data, AI can also carry out more complicated tasks such as evaluating the severity of valvular regurgitant lesions or identifying specific cardiomyopathies such as HCM or cardiac amyloidosis, potentially helping to prevent diagnostic errors.[16,26] A heart failure cardiologist, in situations of diagnostic uncertainty, might benefit from having AI review images or clinical data to support or refute possible diagnoses.[16] For a structural cardiologist, AI could potentially offer insights into a patient's post-procedure survival, an important piece of information to guide shared decision-making.[25] Ultimately, AI may advance a central goal of medicine which is to improve patient health by timely and accurate identification of disease followed by appropriate treatments that consider both the disease and the patient.

AI-guided approaches have limitations. In general, ML algorithms for medical use must have access to a large database of well-curated data that are representative of the pathology they are expected to encounter. AI may be affected by selection bias when training data are insufficiently diverse.[6] For example, note how the accuracy of a DL algorithm for the evaluation of RVEF improved when (re)trained on a more diverse set of scans enriched for RV pathology.[55] Work from both Davies and Chauhan shows how AI algorithms may be confounded when confronted with uncommon pathology not seen regularly in training.[48,49] It is up to the humans using AI to recognize its limitations and to confirm the algorithm's conclusions. Knowing how an AI was trained is important as is knowing if and how the model was externally validated (see **Table 1**). Additionally, there are regulatory requirements that must be met. In the United States, for example, the Food and Drug Administration (FDA) must issue clearance for AI-enabled medical devices, including software, and requires human input so that AI tools are used as clinical decision support.[60]

There have been concerns expressed about the "black box" nature of many AI algorithms wherein an output is generated without an explanation of how the conclusion was reached. This may reduce the health care provider's (and patient) trust in the algorithms. Thus, more recent work such as that by Fahmy and Otaki has explored the concept of explainable AI where the role of different factors in reaching a prediction is noted.[33,58] In the future, the ability of an AI to explain its reasoning may improve clinician trust in the results, especially important for those who are to be responsible for the final clinical decision. Additionally, it is conceivable that explainable AI could some day be hypothesis-generating, analyzing large data sets, and identifying possible new disease mechanisms for future research.

SUMMARY

Cardiac imaging plays a crucial role in the diagnosis and management of heart failure. Given the role that imaging plays in ejection fraction quantification, determination of heart failure etiology, and evaluation of valvular dysfunction, it is crucial that these studies be accurate, reliable, and reproducible. A growing body of research has identified areas where AI can be applied to cardiac imaging. It is likely that future clinical practice will integrate AI in multiple areas, including workflow optimization of imaging laboratories as well as consideration of clinical and imaging parameters to help guide the management of complex heart failure patients.

CLINICS CARE POINTS

- Research has identified promising possible roles for AI in laboratory efficiency, risk stratification, and image analysis.

- In the United States, AI software must be FDA-cleared and function as clinical decision support. Currently available cardiology examples include cardiac chamber quantification.

- When using AI, it is important to understand the nature and limitations of the training data sets.

- The final clinical decision rests with the clinician.

REFERENCES

1. Tsao CW, Aday AW, Almarzooq ZI, et al. Heart disease and stroke statistics-2022 update: a report from the american heart association. Circulation 22 2022;145(8):e153–639.
2. Heidenreich PA, Albert NM, Allen LA, et al. Forecasting the impact of heart failure in the United States: a policy statement from the American Heart Association. Circ Heart Fail 2013;6(3):606–19.
3. Yasmin F, Shah SMI, Naeem A, et al. Artificial intelligence in the diagnosis and detection of heart failure: the past, present, and future. Rev Cardiovasc Med 2021;22(4):1095–113.

4. Ski CF, Thompson DR, Brunner-La Rocca HP. Putting AI at the centre of heart failure care. ESC Heart Fail 2020;7(5):3257–8.

5. Quer G, Arnaout R, Henne M, et al. Machine learning and the future of cardiovascular care: JACc state-of-the-art review. J Am Coll Cardiol 2021;77(3):300–13.

6. Nakamura T, Sasano T. Artificial intelligence and cardiology: current status and perspective. J Cardiol 2022;79(3):326–33.

7. Seetharam K, Min JK. Artificial intelligence and machine learning in cardiovascular imaging. Methodist Debakey Cardiovasc J 2020;16(4):263–71.

8. Kriegeskorte N, Golan T. Neural network models and deep learning. Curr Biol 2019;29(7):R231–6.

9. Romiti S, Vinciguerra M, Saade W, et al. Artificial intelligence (AI) and cardiovascular diseases: an unexpected alliance. Cardiol Res Pract 2020;2020:4972346.

10. Deo RC. Machine learning in medicine. Circulation 2015;132(20):1920–30.

11. Krittanawong C, Zhang H, Wang Z, et al. Artificial intelligence in precision cardiovascular medicine. J Am Coll Cardiol 2017;69(21):2657–64.

12. Krittanawong C, Johnson KW, Rosenson RS, et al. Deep learning for cardiovascular medicine: a practical primer. Eur Heart J 2019;40(25):2058–73.

13. Knackstedt C, Bekkers SC, Schummers G, et al. Fully automated versus standard tracking of left ventricular ejection fraction and longitudinal strain: the FAST-EFs multicenter study. J Am Coll Cardiol 2015;66(13):1456–66.

14. Ouyang D, He B, Ghorbani A, et al. Video-based AI for beat-to-beat assessment of cardiac function. Nature 2020;580(7802):252–6.

15. Li T, Wei B, Cong J, Hong Y, et al. Direct estimation of left ventricular ejection fraction via a cardiac cycle feature learning architecture. Comput Biol Med 2020;118:103659.

16. Zhang J, Gajjala S, Agrawal P, et al. Fully automated echocardiogram interpretation in clinical practice. Circulation 2018;138(16):1623–35.

17. Nagueh SF, Smiseth OA, Appleton CP, et al. Recommendations for the evaluation of left ventricular diastolic function by echocardiography: an update from the american society of echocardiography and the European association of cardiovascular imaging. J Am Soc Echocardiogr 2016;29(4):277–314.

18. Tokodi M, Shrestha S, Bianco C, et al. Interpatient similarities in cardiac function: a platform for personalized cardiovascular medicine. JACC Cardiovasc Imaging 2020;13(5):1119–32.

19. Lancaster MC, Salem Omar AM, Narula S, et al. Phenotypic clustering of left ventricular diastolic function parameters: patterns and prognostic relevance. JACC Cardiovasc Imaging 2019;12(7 Pt 1):1149–61.

20. Pandey A, Kagiyama N, Yanamala N, et al. Deep-learning models for the echocardiographic assessment of diastolic dysfunction. JACC Cardiovasc Imaging 2021;14(10):1887–900.

21. Beecy AN, Bratt A, Yum B, et al. Development of novel machine learning model for right ventricular quantification on echocardiography-A multimodality validation study. Echocardiography 2020;37(5):688–97.

22. Genovese D, Rashedi N, Weinert L, et al. Machine learning-based three-dimensional echocardiographic quantification of right ventricular size and function: validation against cardiac magnetic resonance. J Am Soc Echocardiogr 2019;32(8):969–77.

23. Nedadur R, Wang B, Tsang W. Artificial intelligence for the echocardiographic assessment of valvular heart disease. Heart 2022;108(20):1592–9.

24. Thalappillil R, Datta P, Datta S, et al. Artificial intelligence for the measurement of the aortic valve annulus. J Cardiothorac Vasc Anesth 2020;34(1):65–71.

25. Lachmann M, Rippen E, Schuster T, et al. Subphenotyping of patients with aortic stenosis by unsupervised agglomerative clustering of echocardiographic and hemodynamic data. JACC Cardiovasc Interv 2021;14(19):2127–40.

26. Zhang Q, Liu Y, Mi J, et al. Automatic assessment of mitral regurgitation severity using the mask R-CNN algorithm with color doppler echocardiography images. Comput Math Methods Med 2021;2021:2602688.

27. Chen J, Li H, He G, et al. Automatic 3D mitral valve leaflet segmentation and validation of quantitative measurement. Biomedical Signal Processing and Control 2023;79:104166.

28. Kagiyama N, Toki M, Hara M, et al. Efficacy and accuracy of novel automated mitral valve quantification: three-dimensional transesophageal echocardiographic study. Echocardiography 2016;33(5):756–63.

29. Dabiri Y, Yao J, Mahadevan VS, et al. Mitral valve atlas for artificial intelligence predictions of mitraclip intervention outcomes. Front Cardiovasc Med 2021;8:759675.

30. Miller JM, Rochitte CE, Dewey M, et al. Diagnostic performance of coronary angiography by 64-row CT. N Engl J Med 2008;359(22):2324–36.

31. Arsanjani R, Xu Y, Dey D, et al. Improved accuracy of myocardial perfusion SPECT for detection of coronary artery disease by machine learning in a large population. J Nucl Cardiol 2013;20(4):553–62.

32. Arsanjani R, Dey D, Khachatryan T, et al. Prediction of revascularization after myocardial perfusion SPECT by machine learning in a large population. J Nucl Cardiol 2015;22(5):877–84.

33. Otaki Y, Singh A, Kavanagh P, et al. Clinical deployment of explainable artificial intelligence of SPECT

for diagnosis of coronary artery disease. JACC Cardiovasc Imaging 2022;15(6):1091–102.

34. Pijls NH, De Bruyne B, Peels K, et al. Measurement of fractional flow reserve to assess the functional severity of coronary-artery stenoses. N Engl J Med 1996;334(26):1703–8.

35. Taylor CA, Fonte TA, Min JK. Computational fluid dynamics applied to cardiac computed tomography for noninvasive quantification of fractional flow reserve: scientific basis. J Am Coll Cardiol 2013; 61(22):2233–41.

36. Itu L, Rapaka S, Passerini T, et al. A machine-learning approach for computation of fractional flow reserve from coronary computed tomography. J Appl Physiol 2016;121(1):42–52.

37. Coenen A, Kim YH, Kruk M, et al. Diagnostic accuracy of a machine-learning approach to coronary computed tomographic angiography-based fractional flow reserve: result from the MACHINE consortium. Circ Cardiovasc Imaging 2018;11(6): e007217.

38. Choi AD, Marques H, Kumar V, et al. CT Evaluation by Artificial Intelligence for Atherosclerosis, Stenosis and Vascular Morphology (CLARIFY): A Multi-center, international study. J Cardiovasc Comput Tomogr 2021;15(6):470–6.

39. Griffin WF, Choi AD, Riess JS, et al. AI evaluation of stenosis on coronary Ct angiography, comparison with quantitative coronary angiography and fractional flow reserve: a CREDENCE trial substudy. JACC Cardiovasc Imaging 2022. https://doi.org/10.1016/j.jcmg.2021.10.020.

40. Lipkin I, Telluri A, Kim Y, et al. Coronary CTA with AI-QCT interpretation: comparison with myocardial perfusion imaging for detection of obstructive stenosis using invasive angiography as reference standard. AJR Am J Roentgenol 2022;219(3):407–19.

41. Bellenger NG, Burgess MI, Ray SG, et al. Comparison of left ventricular ejection fraction and volumes in heart failure by echocardiography, radionuclide ventriculography and cardiovascular magnetic resonance; are they interchangeable? Eur Heart J 2000; 21(16):1387–96.

42. Grothues F, Smith GC, Moon JC, et al. Comparison of interstudy reproducibility of cardiovascular magnetic resonance with two-dimensional echocardiography in normal subjects and in patients with heart failure or left ventricular hypertrophy. Am J Cardiol 2002;90(1):29–34.

43. Addetia K, Bhave NM, Tabit CE, et al. Sample size and cost analysis for pulmonary arterial hypertension drug trials using various imaging modalities to assess right ventricular size and function end points. Circ Cardiovasc Imaging 2014;7(1):115–24.

44. Heidenreich PA, Bozkurt B, Aguilar D, et al. 2022 AHA/ACC/HFSA guideline for the management of heart failure: executive summary: a report of the American College of Cardiology/American heart association joint committee on clinical practice guidelines. Circulation 2022;145(18):e876–94.

45. Bernard O, Lalande A, Zotti C, et al. Deep learning techniques for automatic MRI cardiac multi-structures segmentation and diagnosis: is the problem solved? IEEE Trans Med Imaging 2018;37(11): 2514–25.

46. Bai W, Sinclair M, Tarroni G, et al. Automated cardiovascular magnetic resonance image analysis with fully convolutional networks. J Cardiovasc Magn Reson 2018;20(1):65.

47. Tao Q, Yan W, Wang Y, et al. Deep learning-based method for fully automatic quantification of left ventricle function from cine MR images: a multivendor, multicenter study. Radiology 2019;290(1): 81–8.

48. Davies RH, Augusto JB, Bhuva A, et al. Precision measurement of cardiac structure and function in cardiovascular magnetic resonance using machine learning. J Cardiovasc Magn Reson 2022;24(1):16.

49. Chauhan D, Anyanwu E, Goes J, et al. Comparison of machine learning and deep learning for view identification from cardiac magnetic resonance images. Clin Imaging 2022;82:121–6.

50. Clarke CJ, Gurka MJ, Norton PT, et al. Assessment of the accuracy and reproducibility of RV volume measurements by CMR in congenital heart disease. JACC Cardiovasc Imaging 2012;5(1):28–37.

51. Mooij CF, de Wit CJ, Graham DA, et al. Reproducibility of MRI measurements of right ventricular size and function in patients with normal and dilated ventricles. J Magn Reson Imaging 2008;28(1): 67–73.

52. Grothues F, Moon JC, Bellenger NG, et al. Interstudy reproducibility of right ventricular volumes, function, and mass with cardiovascular magnetic resonance. Am Heart J 2004;147(2):218–23.

53. Backhaus SJ, Staab W, Steinmetz M, et al. Fully automated quantification of biventricular volumes and function in cardiovascular magnetic resonance: applicability to clinical routine settings. J Cardiovasc Magn Reson 2019;21(1):24.

54. Wang S, Patel H, Miller T, et al. AI based CMR assessment of biventricular function: clinical significance of intervendor variability and measurement errors. JACC Cardiovasc Imaging 2022;15(3): 413–27.

55. Wang S, Chauhan D, Patel H, et al. Assessment of right ventricular size and function from cardiovascular magnetic resonance images using artificial intelligence. J Cardiovasc Magn Reson 2022;24(1):27.

56. Fahmy AS, Rausch J, Neisius U, et al. Automated cardiac MR scar quantification in hypertrophic cardiomyopathy using deep convolutional neural networks. JACC Cardiovasc Imaging Dec 2018; 11(12):1917–8.

57. Zhang Q, Burrage MK, Lukaschuk E, et al. Toward replacing late gadolinium enhancement with artificial intelligence virtual native enhancement for gadolinium-free cardiovascular magnetic resonance tissue characterization in hypertrophic cardiomyopathy. Circulation 2021;144(8):589–99.

58. Fahmy AS, Csecs I, Arafati A, et al. An explainable machine learning approach reveals prognostic significance of right ventricular dysfunction in nonischemic cardiomyopathy. JACC Cardiovasc Imaging 2022;15(5):766–79.

59. Dawes TJW, de Marvao A, Shi W, et al. Machine learning of three-dimensional right ventricular motion enables outcome prediction in pulmonary hypertension: a cardiac MR imaging study. Radiology 2017;283(2):381–90.

60. United States Food and Drug Administration. Artificial Intelligence and Machine Learning (AI/ML)-Enabled Medical Devices. 2022. https://www.fda.gov/medical-devices/software-medical-device-samd/artificial-intelligence-and-machine-learning-aiml-enabled-medical-devices. Accessed December 13, 2022.

UNITED STATES POSTAL SERVICE ®

Statement of Ownership, Management, and Circulation
(All Periodicals Publications Except Requester Publications)

1. Publication Title	2. Publication Number		3. Filing Date
HEART FAILURE CLINICS	025 – 055		9/18/2023

4. Issue Frequency	5. Number of Issues Published Annually	6. Annual Subscription Price
JAN, APR, JUL, OCT	4	$291.00

7. Complete Mailing Address of Known Office of Publication (Not printer) (Street, city, county, state, and ZIP+4®)

ELSEVIER INC.
230 Park Avenue, Suite 800
New York, NY 10169

Contact Person: Malathi Samayan
Telephone (Include area code): 91-44-4299-4507

8. Complete Mailing Address of Headquarters or General Business Office of Publisher (Not printer)

ELSEVIER INC.
230 Park Avenue, Suite 800
New York, NY 10169

9. Full Names and Complete Mailing Addresses of Publisher, Editor, and Managing Editor (Do not leave blank)

Publisher (Name and complete mailing address)

Dolores Meloni, ELSEVIER INC.
1600 JOHN F KENNEDY BLVD. SUITE 1600
PHILADELPHIA, PA 19103-2899

Editor (Name and complete mailing address)

JOANNA GASCOINE, ELSEVIER INC.
1600 JOHN F KENNEDY BLVD. SUITE 1600
PHILADELPHIA, PA 19103-2899

Managing Editor (Name and complete mailing address)

PATRICK MANLEY, ELSEVIER INC.
1600 JOHN F KENNEDY BLVD. SUITE 1600
PHILADELPHIA, PA 19103-2899

10. Owner (Do not leave blank. If the publication is owned by a corporation, give the name and address of the corporation immediately followed by the names and addresses of all stockholders owning or holding 1 percent or more of the total amount of stock. If not owned by a corporation, give the names and addresses of the individual owners. If owned by a partnership or other unincorporated firm, give its name and address as well as those of each individual owner. If the publication is published by a nonprofit organization, give its name and address.)

Full Name	Complete Mailing Address
WHOLLY OWNED SUBSIDIARY OF REED/ELSEVIER, US HOLDINGS	1600 JOHN F KENNEDY BLVD. SUITE 1600 PHILADELPHIA, PA 19103-2899

11. Known Bondholders, Mortgagees, and Other Security Holders Owning or Holding 1 Percent or More of Total Amount of Bonds, Mortgages, or Other Securities. If none, check box ☐ None

Full Name	Complete Mailing Address
N/A	

12. Tax Status (For completion by nonprofit organizations authorized to mail at nonprofit rates) (Check one)
The purpose, function, and nonprofit status of this organization and the exempt status for federal income tax purposes:

☒ Has Not Changed During Preceding 12 Months
☐ Has Changed During Preceding 12 Months (Publisher must submit explanation of change with this statement)

PS Form **3526**, July 2014 (Page 1 of 4 (see instructions page 4)] PSN: 7530-01-000-9931   PRIVACY NOTICE: See our privacy policy on www.usps.com.

---

13. Publication Title	14. Issue Date for Circulation Data Below
HEART FAILURE CLINICS	JULY 2023

15. Extent and Nature of Circulation			Average No. Copies Each Issue During Preceding 12 Months	No. Copies of Single Issue Published Nearest to Filing Date
a. Total Number of Copies (Net press run)			92	72
b. Paid Circulation (By Mail and Outside the Mail)	(1)	Mailed Outside-County Paid Subscriptions Stated on PS Form 3541 (Include paid distribution above nominal rate, advertiser's proof copies, and exchange copies)	38	36
	(2)	Mailed In-County Paid Subscriptions Stated on PS Form 3541 (Include paid distribution above nominal rate, advertiser's proof copies, and exchange copies)	0	0
	(3)	Paid Distribution Outside the Mails Including Sales Through Dealers and Carriers, Street Vendors, Counter Sales, and Other Paid Distribution Outside USPS®	43	24
	(4)	Paid Distribution by Other Classes of Mail Through the USPS (e.g., First-Class Mail®)	10	11
c. Total Paid Distribution (Sum of 15b (1), (2), (3), and (4))		▶	91	71
d. Free or Nominal Rate Distribution (By Mail and Outside the Mail)	(1)	Free or Nominal Rate Outside-County Copies Included on PS Form 3541	0	0
	(2)	Free or Nominal Rate In-County Copies Included on PS Form 3541	0	0
	(3)	Free or Nominal Rate Copies Mailed at Other Classes Through the USPS (e.g., First-Class Mail)	0	0
	(4)	Free or Nominal Rate Distribution Outside the Mail (Carriers or other means)	1	1
e. Total Free or Nominal Rate Distribution (Sum of 15d (1), (2), (3) and (4))		▶	1	1
f. Total Distribution (Sum of 15c and 15e)		▶	92	72
g. Copies not Distributed (See Instructions to Publishers #4 (page 83))		▶	0	0
h. Total (Sum of 15f and g)		▶	92	72
i. Percent Paid (15c divided by 15f times 100)			98.91%	98.61%

* If you are claiming electronic copies, go to line 16 on page 3. If you are not claiming electronic copies, skip to line 17 on page 3.

16. Electronic Copy Circulation		Average No. Copies Each Issue During Preceding 12 Months	No. Copies of Single Issue Published Nearest to Filing Date
a. Paid Electronic Copies	▶		
b. Total Paid Print Copies (Line 15c) + Paid Electronic Copies (Line 16a)	▶		
c. Total Print Distribution (Line 15f) + Paid Electronic Copies (Line 16a)	▶		
d. Percent Paid (Both Print & Electronic Copies) (16b divided by 16c × 100)	▶		

☒ I certify that 80% of all my distributed copies (electronic and print) are paid above a nominal price.

17. Publication of Statement of Ownership

☒ If the publication is a general publication, publication of this statement is required. Will be printed
in the OCTOBER 2023 issue of this publication. ☐ Publication not required.

18. Signature and Title of Editor, Publisher, Business Manager, or Owner	Date
Malathi Samayan Malathi Samayan - Distribution Controller	9/18/2023

I certify that all information furnished on this form is true and complete. I understand that anyone who furnishes false or misleading information on this form or who omits material or information requested on the form may be subject to criminal sanctions (including fines and imprisonment) and/or civil sanctions (including civil penalties).

PS Form **3526**, July 2014 (Page 3 of 4)   PRIVACY NOTICE: See our privacy policy on www.usps.com.

Printed and bound by CPI Group (UK) Ltd, Croydon, CR0 4YY

03/10/2024

01040367-0009